Living With Cancer

Living With Cancer

Meditations on Patience and Love

Melody Kee Smith and Richard Smith

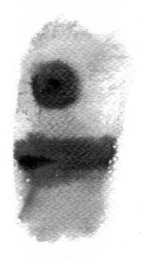

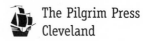 The Pilgrim Press
Cleveland

I dedicate this book to my loving and steadfast companion on the journey, my husband Richard. I truly could not do this life without him! With humble and heartfelt gratitude, I also dedicate this book to all my care-givers, professional and personal, and family and friends, some of whose stories fill the pages of this book. And to you, the reader, whose own stories could fill a book, thanks for relating to mine. Finally, I dedicate this book to my God, the Creator, Redeemer, Sustainer, and Healer of all life. To God be the glory!

Melody Kee Smith

The Pilgrim Press, 700 Prospect Avenue, Cleveland, Ohio 44115-1100
pilgrimpress.com
© 2001 by Melody Kee Smith and Richard Smith

Printed in the United States of America on acid-free paper

06   05   04   03   02   01   5   4   3   2   1

Library of Congress Cataloging-in-Publication Data

Smith, Melody Kee, 1947–
    Living with cancer : meditations on patience and love /
  Melody Kee Smith and Richard Smith.
      p.   cm.
    ISBN 0-8298-1436-1
    1. Cancer—Patients—Prayer-books and devotions—English.
I. Smith, Richard (Richard A.), 1947–   II. Title.

BV4910.33 .S55   2001
242'.4—dc21

2001044607

contents

preface

IN AUGUST OF 1987 my wife-to-be was diagnosed with advanced metastatic breast cancer. Following a radical mastectomy and a series of chemotherapy treatments, she (and by extension, I) remained cancer-free for nine years. We gratefully celebrated the conclusion of the fifth of those nine, knowing that she had passed the "magic moment" of statistical triumph over this disease. We were stunned to learn of the Big C's return in 1996, and we have been fighting it ever since, keeping it at bay as best we can, she on the inside, me on the outside.

Over the past few years, which have involved chemotherapy, radiation, the side-effects of each, and the fatigue and fear that come with struggling against such as relentless foe, Melody has found strength and purpose through a combination of two qualities she possesses in extraordinary abundance: her extroversion and her introspection. Drawing from her contact with and love of others, and reflecting daily upon her experiences through journaling, she came to a realization that her journey might have parallels to the challenges others face in dealing with cancer—or, indeed, any life-threatening illness.

In reviewing her daily meditations, she found that they lent themselves to questions for reflection and opportunities for prayer. Along the lines of the latter, she asked if I would be willing to write

a brief prayer in response to each of the meditations she has offered here. I am honored to do so. I am honored to be associated
with this gem of encouragement. I am honored, beyond my ability to say or show, to be partner to a woman with this kind of
courage, this much love, this ability for self-reflection, this depth
of patient faith. I thank God that my wife-to-be is my wife still.

The Reverend Richard Allan Smith

author's note

I TRUST THAT YOU, the reader, will find some comfort and challenge in these pages. We all need both in our lives. In the past
year, I have continued to be comforted by love and support from
family, friends, and God. I have also been challenged by several,
thankfully minor, recurrences of cancer. At those times, I go to my
writing and my Creator as a source of strength and hope. I believe
I will ultimately be healed of this disease, to have Life abundant.
I believe you can, too. God bless you and keep you!

Love and Patience,
Melody Kee Smith

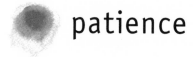 # patience

IN SOME WAYS, this has been the hardest year of all for me in my nearly fourteen-year struggle with cancer. After my last chemotherapy, I developed a hoarseness and weakness of my voice that is still present. At first, I was treated for asthma and allergies with little or no results. Finally, an ENT (ear, nose, and throat) doctor diagnosed it as a paralysis of my left vocal cord, which may or may not be permanent. Since then, I have been in speech therapy with slow, minimal progress to date. It has been frustrating and discouraging for me. I miss being able to speak normally and especially to sing at all. I have alternated between depression, anger, hopelessness, and a fierce determination to get better no matter what it takes.

· What unusual side effect of cancer has affected you the most? How do you deal with frustration and discouragement?
· What do you think might be hardest for you to lose to cancer?

Keep music in our hearts, God, even when the notes will not come to our lips. When our voices will not be heard, let the angels join in a chorus of hope. Amen.

PART OF LEARNING to deal with this "loss of voice" is learning to compensate in the ways I use my voice. My speech therapist is retraining me to talk "lower and slower." I have also found, thanks to Richard's Internet capabilities, a voice amplifier that helps me to project without straining. It is much like a fanny pack with headphones attached. Its trade name is "Chattervox" but I have renamed it "Chatty Cathy" like the doll of many years ago. To me, this is a more personal and user-friendly concept. Almost like an alter ego.

· Have you ever had to compensate for loss of an ability? How was that for you?
· What function has cancer taken away from you that you miss?
· Is there an "alter ego" in your life?

Grace us, O God, with the memories of childhood that can enrich our lives as adults. Let the child that comes to you at times be our own selves. Amen.

I HAD AN EXAMPLE of God's perfect timing today. When I went to get the mail, there was a thick packet from UCC Pilgrim Press addressed to Richard and me. We had sent them our manuscript for *Living With Cancer* quite awhile ago and had just about given up. I was sure they were returning it to us with a rejection letter. Was I ever surprised and overwhelmed to find them offering us a book contract! This, at a time when I had lost heart about ever having a voice again. Now, it seems, I have a new voice, that of communicating in writing as a way of reaching out to help others to heal.

- What's the best surprise you've ever received in the mail?
- Have you ever felt like you "lost your voice" (or your heart)?
- If you could write a book, what would it be called?

God, you do not always come to us when we ask, but you are always right on time. Amen.

LATELY, I HAVE HAD TO ADMIT what a "control freak" I am about my time. Not that I'm so prompt, because I'm not; rather, it has more to do with how I rigidly make a schedule and stick to it. In this regard, I can be rather brutal on myself and others close to me. I hate to waste time and I especially hate not to know in advance what I'm doing when. Thus, it was an interesting learning experience for me to come home for a visit without all my time slots filled in. I had contacted some folks but a lot of plans were indefinite. For me, it was an exercise in trusting that I would get together with those I most needed to see—and that would be determined when I got there . . . All I had to do was believe things would work out as they were supposed to . . .

- How do you operate in relation to time schedules?
- Have you ever felt you had to let go of managing your time and just let things develop?
- Do you believe that things happen as they're meant to?

We need a sense of Sabbath, God, a time without time's constraints and controls. May we have the peaceful grace it takes to let even one day, one hour, one moment be yours and not ours. Amen.

People don't ever realize how small gestures they make can have such a big impact. Today, after church, one of the women, Elaine, handed me a magazine. She explained that she remembered me telling her that I was getting into gardening but that I had a lot of shade in my yard so it was a challenge. The magazine had an article in it on flowers for shade gardens. I am touched deeply by this gesture. First of all, I hardly know this woman. Second, how sweet of her to remember our conversation. But, most of all, I reflect with a lump in my throat, she must think I'm going to be around for a while to enjoy the flowers I plant. Her hope gives me hope to continue planting.

- Have there been "small gestures" of kindness done to you recently? How did this feel?
- What in your life gives you the sense that you will "go on ..."?
- Draw a garden you'd like to have.

Your promise to us, O God, is that we will each rest under our own vine and fig tree. May that promise extend to our peonies and roses as well. Amen.

In every church, there is at least one (and usually several) individuals of which it is said, "I don't think we could get along without . . . " In our present church, the person most often mentioned in this regard is Dorly Brunner. Dorly is an incredibly skilled and energetic woman of Swiss origin. Among other things, Dorly is head of our Mission Board, plans, shops for, and oversees the making of our Soup Kitchen meals, organizes our funeral receptions, coordinates our Thanksgiving baskets, does our church recycling, organizes our Crop Walk, etc. etc. etc. (not to mention all she does for the community and individuals outside our church!). This morning at church, however, Dorly did the best thing she's ever done for me. She let me see myself by being a mirror for me. While chatting with me during coffee hour, she listened to me, then intervened with "Now, Melody, don't you think you're doing just a little too much?" In response, all I could do was smile. To her credit, she blushed and smiled in return!

- Is there a "Dorly" in your church, synagogue, temple, workplace, neighborhood, etc.?
- Can you relate, in any way, to this person? Why or why not?
- When you're "caught" by your own words, are you able to admit it? Any instances that come to mind?

Enable us, O God, to use all the gifts you have given us, and to be open to the gifts of others being shared in our lives. Amen.

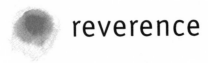

reverence

I FINALLY REACH my brother Dan by phone after trying for several days. I've been wanting to let him know the good news that I'm finished with my radiation. He is oddly noncommittal in his response. In fact, I reflect to myself, he's not been very present for me throughout this round of cancer. I begin to silently nurture old resentments and hurts (unfortunately, all too typical of me!). He must sense this, because after a bit more idle conversation, he says to me, "Mel, I never doubted you'd be OK. You've been healed of cancer. God has work for you to do yet. You have a ministry of healing." He says this with such conviction! My brother is firmly rooted in his fundamentalist, charismatic Christianity. I, on the other hand, have a more questioning and evolving faith. I believe there is room in God's heart for both of us. I can only hope and pray that Dan does, too. He is my only brother and I want to be with him wherever "there" is despite our many differences. I believe God wants this, too.

· How have your brother(s) and sister(s) been with you in the course of your cancer? What do you need and want that you're not getting from them? What has helped you most?
· Do you have philosophical/spiritual differences with your sibling(s)? How does this affect your contacts and conversations with them?
· Do you think God has "favorite children"? (Be honest!)

Our hardest hurts are all too often between us and those closest to us. Help us to get past the old patterns and resentments to some new day of brotherly and sisterly love. Amen.

THERE IS A POPULAR SONG by Lionel Ritchie, part of which goes ". . . that's why I'm easy—easy like Sunday morning." What a joke! Being in the ministry is anything but "easy" on Sunday mornings. There's always one more detail or person to whom one must attend. So often I end up arriving at church looking and feeling frazzled. This morning, during my devotional time, the fourth commandment comes to mind. I decide to consciously try to slow myself down this Sunday morning—and to truly "remember the sabbath day, and keep it holy." As part of this, I take the time to walk to church instead of doing "one more thing" and roaring into the parking lot at the last minute. It is a pleasant, soft early summer morning—lots of colorful bulbs are still flowering, but very few people are out. On the way, I even stop to chat with a neighbor I've never met. As the church bells ring, I stroll up to the door, humming a favorite hymn. I feel positively "easy"!

· Have your worship experiences been "easy" or "hard" for you? Why?
· What does it mean to you to "see the sacred in the ordinary"? Has this ever happened for you?
· Be aware of something unique in the ordinary events of today. Find some unique way to recognize this.

Grant us the faithfulness to observe the sabbath and the sabbatical moments that will be offered to us this day. Enable us to remember how to rest. Amen.

TODAY, THOUGH IT IS A SATURDAY, we have a baptism at church. It is late afternoon and the sunlight is gentle and warm, the baby beautiful, the family proud. There is a special quality to being in church when one is not "supposed to" be there. It is as if we are all invited to a surprise party in the church! As I sit, sharing this sacred time, I realize I am at peace. How wonderful it is to be in the moment, to feel alive and whole! I wonder if this disease is not making me more aware of the uniqueness in the ordinary events of life. Just for now, I am thankful that I have been enabled to "see" because of my cancer.

· Remember a baptism that meant something special to you and why that was.
· Have you ever been surprised by feeling "at peace"? How and when did this occur?
· Note the ways in which you can "see" better because of the cancer.

May we have the vision to see all the sacramental events and actions and people of this day, O God. Renew and refresh us through what we see. Amen.

I WORK PART-TIME as a social worker for Hospice Home Health Care—a job some say I shouldn't have as a cancer survivor currently "in recurrence." However, I believe I am supposed to be doing this, right here and now. It is a ministry of healing and I get so much more back than I give! The patients and their families so often teach and inspire me. I am simply a fellow guide and comforter on the path we all take from life to death to life again. It is an honor and a blessing to serve not only from education and training but by virtue of personal experience. So today, on Saturday, when I am called to an emergency visit, it is OK. It makes my Saturday sacred. A true sabbath. After my visit, I sit, sipping iced tea with Paul and Carol, good neighbor friends, in their backyard, thinking how good it is to be alive (for however long) . . .

- Are you filling more than one role in your life right now (in addition to surviving cancer)? How are these roles fitting together—or not?
- What do you need to have more of a sense of the "sacred" in your life?
- In what ways might you make more time for "sabbaths" right now (today, even)?

Remind us, O God, that death is a part of life, and that all life is sacred. Let us therefore love life more, and fear death less. Amen.

I GO TO VISIT AURORA, one of my hospice patients. She is a petite, attractive, eighty-year-old French Canadian woman who is frail of body but strong of spirit. Today, though, the cancer has both body and spirit down and in bed. She is really too tired to talk much, drifting off in midsentence despite her desire to be pleasant and polite. I squeeze her hand gently, stroke her brow, and leave her to much-needed rest. Earlier, though, we had spoken of the afterlife. She had told me that, although she wasn't exactly sure what it would be like, it was definitely something to look forward to and not to fear. Such words of strength and courage from one so close to the end of "life" as we know it! I wonder, would I be as brave if I truly believed that this was "it" for me? Asking this question makes me realize—to my surprise and delight—that I don't believe that the cancer is going to get me—not this time, at least . . .

- Can you recall being with someone who was in the last stages of dying and basically nonverbal? How did you feel?
- What are your thoughts and beliefs about an afterlife? (Draw a picture if it's easier to express.)
- Ask yourself—honestly—do you fear dying? In what sense?

For the remarkable intuitions of life, we are grateful to you, Victor over death. Amen.

SOME OLDER COUPLES give me hope for what it will be like to grow older and still be in love. One of these is Jan and Don Thatcher, married fifty years this year, and sparkling with zest for life and each other. Sadly, this year Don developed prostrate cancer, which did not respond to treatment and has since spread to his brain. Throughout this frightening and discouraging process, they have maintained faith in one another and in God. They have inspired and touched all of us who know and love them. They never fail to inquire about my health—even in the darkest of times for them. Today, Don asked Richard to come and give him and Jan communion, as he felt the end was near. He also asked that I be present with them. As we stood, holding hands and praying around Don's bedside, there was such undeniable love around and among us that death truly felt dwarfed. The peace of God was present in a most palpable way. "Perfect love casts out fear."

- What kind of "older couple" do you think you'll be? (or are ... or have been ...)
- If you're not part of a couple, who in your life is closest to you during this time? Have you ever had a "soul mate"?
- When is the last time you've truly felt the peace of God in a tangible sense?

Grant us the courage to reach out for the hand we need, call out for the voice we long to hear, seek the presence of the ones we want by our side. Let us be strong enough to need. Amen.

ONE OF THE TAPES that my brother Dan has been playing a lot while I've been here has a song called "Extravagant Love" about the love of God for each of us. To me, my brother embodies this extravagant love in his work with the folks he serves in his storefront church. Nothing is too small or unimportant for his time and attentions. One Sunday evening after a service at which he preached, he called for people to come forward who wanted prayers to deliver them from a fear that had its grip on their lives. I immediately knew that I needed prayer for the fear that grips my life by the name of "cancer." So, with some trepidation, I went forward and had my brother pray with me. I was moved to tears, as was he, but afterwards I felt lighter and more hopeful.

· Have you ever experienced "extravagant love"?
· Is there a fear that has its grip on your life?
· Recall a time when someone prayed with you ...

Thou, who cares for the lilies of the fields and the birds of the air: will you show some extravagant, outrageous love to us today? Will we see it? May we? Amen.

Today was Music Sunday in church—and a good time was had by all! This is the Sunday we get to let loose, be creative, and maybe even be a little bit offbeat (probably not a term I should use in this instance!). We had choirs of all ages, even a bell choir, all kinds of instrumentalists, and plenty of enthusiastic congregational support. Now, I'm not sure where I stand on the issue of all this clapping in church—after all, it is worship and praise, not performance. But I do admit I could picture God tapping his feet and nodding her head to the rhythm. It was a lovely gathering of God's people with not a moment to focus on being sick—only on being—thanks *be* to God!

- Reflect on what it means to you to "make a joyful noise" unto God.
- Are you willing to experiment with different ways of "being" in church? Like what, for example? If not, why not?
- Find something to clap your hands (and maybe even stomp your feet) about today.

Be the rhythm of our lives, the melody of the angels, the harmony of the heavens; and let us be the joyful noise of God. Amen.

happiness

ORDINARILY, I LOVE TO LAUGH. As a girl, I spent a lot of time giggling. Lately, with the cancer back, I haven't laughed as much even though my minister husband, Richard, has a great sense of timing and could moonlight as a standup comic (wouldn't that pack them into the church?!). This afternoon, though, I received something in the mail that made me fairly howl with delight. I was absolutely gleeful. My childhood friend, Sheila, sent me a card she'd made on her computer. It was a picture of me (from twenty-five years ago) next to Sean Connery. He is both Sheila's and my favorite actor; actually, to tell the truth, we're both rather obsessed with him. And no, I have never met him — and most likely never will. This was all Sheila's way of cheering me up by catering to my romantic midlife fantasies. And it worked! Even if we don't meet, it's nice to know he cares . . . and even nicer to be understood and accepted by someone who knew me when. God is like that with each one of us — caring for us no matter what age or condition.

- Who is your "idol"? Have you ever had a "crush" on someone? As an adult? (Be honest!)
- Who or what makes you laugh? When is the last time you really laughed? Find something to laugh about today — and "let 'er rip!"
- Does God have a sense of humor? How do you know this?

Thank you, God, for the gifts of imagination and of lifelong friends; for fantasy and reality; for the meetings of the two. Amen.

On the last day of radiation, I am elated to be finished! I try hard not to gloat about it to my newfound "buddies" in the waiting room, as some of them aren't going to be finished for a month or more. Yet, as I toss my last (I pray) hospital gown in the bin and round the corner to the outside waiting room, I feel like I could fairly float—I'm so relieved! As I pass the receptionist's desk to get my next token for the patient parking lot (because I will be having follow-up appointments upstairs), I stop to bid her farewell, since I hope not to return to this department again. She responds with enthusiasm for me but says, "I'll miss your warm smile every morning . . . " This surprises me—I didn't know I had been smiling—but it pleases me as well. To be seen makes my day. As God sees each one of us every day.

- Write about your last day of treatment if it's occurred; if not, write about what you think it will be like . . .
- Notice yourself smiling "for no reason at all." If you don't, try it and see how it feels.
- Is there someone or something about the experience of cancer treatment that you (will) miss? Why?

Look on us with kindness, Loving God, and may we give evidence of joy when we are seen. Amen.

Like my mom, I am very aware of my clothing (and everyone else's!). From her, I learned that clothes must complement, coordinate, and, above all, be appropriate to the occasion. Thus, I often change my clothing (and accessories) several times a day. It's kind of a hobby of mine—rather like playing "dress up." This evening, at a church function, I got "caught" by a couple of women in our congregation. It was the third time I'd seen them today at various church gatherings—and the third different outfit I'd had on! The two women are sisters, very close and devoted to one another and to our church. One of them, Carol, said with a twinkle in her eye, "Melody—isn't this the third outfit I've seen you in today?" What could I say? Her sister, Faye, also with a twinkle, responded, "Yes, I think it is—but isn't it just perfect?" My mother would have smiled, which is exactly what I did.

· How does your style of dressing express your sense of yourself? If it doesn't, would you like to change it?
· Do you remember playing "dress up" as a child? Describe (or draw) your favorite outfit.
· Which one of the sisters do you most resemble? How do you feel about this?

May the child in each of us come forth this day, Lord. Help us again to have a playful, loving, faithful joy of life. Amen.

WHILE IN BOSTON to get a second opinion, Richard and I have time to kill before our appointment. Instead of focusing on why we're there, we decide to distract ourselves by "playing tourist." Boston is one of the best places to do this and we do it with gusto. Not only are there historic places to explore—most notably the stops on the Freedom Trail—but lots of colorful urban life to experience. Our favorite thing is to wander and discover—"the more aimlessly the better" is our motto! After our appointment, we go to an Italian restaurant recommended by the doctor. It is fearfully expensive but terribly romantic so we let ourselves enjoy it for what it is. "Whoever thought going to a doctor could be so much fun?" we kid each other. Who indeed?!

- What, in your life, provides a "distraction" from your disease?
- Do you ever have times you "wander aimlessly" (on purpose, that is!)? If not, would you like to?
- When's the last time you "played tourist" or did something spontaneous and perhaps a bit extravagant? How was it?

O God, do not let the real fears of our lives blind us to the possibilities of joy that surround us. Help us today to cherish a pleasure of life. Amen.

ONE OF THE THINGS that has kept both Richard and me going through all the changes in our ten years together is our sense of humor. Quirky. Bizarre. Absurd. Black . . . but humor nonetheless. Another thing that has kept us going strong despite all our struggles is our wonderful sex life. Quite wonderful, in fact. When the two of these factors converge, it is the best of times for us. One such unlikely convergence took place during the radiation treatments. When I went to get "marked" for radiation, Richard teased me about my glowing in the dark. Because of his love for me and our passion for one another, I rather like the image of a tattooed lady . . . and I must admit, there are times we definitely "glow in the dark"!

- How has your humor helped you deal with this illness?
- What part do sexuality and sensuality play in your present life?
- Reflect on times you felt you may have "glowed in the dark."

Lord, let us light it up one more time! Amen!

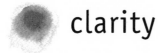 # clarity

IN THE MIDST of uncertainty and fear, good news comes to us. My son Josh was fifteen when we moved from the Midwest to the East so my husband could pastor a church here. It was a most devastating loss for Josh, from which he is still recovering. Today, though, I attended his induction into Spanish Honor Society at school. Afterward, I learned he'd found his first job! Of course, I was a pretty proud parent—but even more so, pleased that he was getting on with his life in a positive way. And—just for a little while—I forgot about my own health. Especially at times when we're struggling with hard issues, we need to remember to stop and savor whatever successes life brings, however small or large. I know at such times God celebrates with us!

· What "good news," however small, has come to you during this time?
· How can you remind yourself to look for what is good?
· What might you do today to celebrate with God?

For the little victories of life that can more than equal the giant tragedies, we give you thanks, our God. Help us to be mindful of "the little things" that make for life. Amen.

THIS MORNING I met with the oncology social worker at her request to convey my perceptions of what went wrong on my first day of treatment. I had already met with the head nurse, who was very sympathetic and sensitive. Today I asked a friend, Lee, to join us, as she is very clear-thinking and assertive. Not only were we able to share openly and feel heard, but we actually got to a place of brainstorming together on ways to improve the system of communication between patients and staff. The social worker was most receptive and affirming—so much so that Lee and I left there discussing setting up possible workshops for local hospitals and clinics. Talk about empowering! Again, I was reminded of how often positive change has a negative catalyst—as is so often the case in our spiritual development. I guess if God doesn't give up on me, I won't either!

· If you're feeling frustrated by "the system" in this process, what can you do to get some satisfaction for yourself?
· Can you see ways in which things could be improved by those delivering your health care?
· Who or what do you need to help you approach these systems or individuals?

Rejection + confrontation + betrayal + denial + crucifixion = resurrection. Amen.

IT IS MEMORIAL DAY and that usually means a picnic. Today is no exception, thanks to Marty and Paul, a generous church couple, who invite us to their home. Gratefully, since we are not gathering until late afternoon, I have most of the day to myself. Wow! What a heady feeling that is! I cycle through all my "shoulds" list, which is, of course, endless. Then I settle down to a "want to" list, which is slowly becoming easier. Since my recurrence, I seem more able to focus on the "essentials"—on what is really important and life-giving. Today, I choose to spend time thinking about family members and close friends who have died—especially my mom and dad. What loving yet imperfect people they were! So very human! Suddenly, I feel them most keenly with me—an integral part of my healing. Remembering heals . . .

· Do you struggle with "want tos" and "shoulds"? Just for today, focus on the "want tos" and see what that feels like. At the end of the day, write what it was like here …
· What lessons have you learned (and continue to learn) from imperfect people (perhaps even your own parents)? How can this help you in your own parenting?
· Are there memories that you need to have "healed"? Name them here …

Sometimes, God, we need the healing of our memories; other times we need our memories to heal our present. Heal us, we pray, at the place of our need. Amen.

BEFORE BEGINNING the radiation therapy, my oncologist, Dr. Susan Rabinowe, sent me to see an orthopedist, Dr. Yanopulos. Her concern was whether the bones in my hip were strong enough to withstand the radiation without fracturing. If not, I might have to have a pin or, worse, an artificial hip replacement before proceeding with treatment. In church, I mentioned this to a friend, Laura, who offered to accompany me, as she is an occupational therapist. I felt relieved not only because she would know the questions to ask but because Laura has such a warm, sunny spirit. That day in the office, I knew I was right to include her.

Both Richard and I were nervous, on edge, and she helped bridge the gap between us and the doctor. He responded well to her concern and knowledge—and best of all, the news was good: no prior surgery was necessary! In a way, it helped me to look forward to the radiation as "the lesser of two evils." Even more, it reminded me that I don't have to go through these appointments alone. I can call on the goodwill and good judgment of friends like Laura. God doesn't intend for us to bear the load all by ourselves.

· What do you go through when you're about to consult yet another specialist?
· Are there people in your life who might be able to help you deal better with these appointments? Make a list of them and decide to ask just one of them to accompany you next time.
· Now—ask yourself why it's so hard to even contemplate doing this (much less acting on it!).

Help us to know not only the limitations of ourselves, but the talents and skills of others. Help us to reach out and accept the love that is offered to us. Help us, O God, to be helped. Amen.

IN SOME WAYS, I am not an easy patient to care for. Partly this is because I ask so many questions and partly because I require a lot of TLC (tender loving care). My oncologist, Dr. Susan Rabinowe, was perfectly fine with the first of these—but not at all sure what to do about the second. She is very well-trained and informed but not a "warm fuzzy" until you get to know her. At one point, I was close to switching to another doctor because of the rather clinical way in which she informed me about my recurrence. After meeting with her to talk it over, I changed my mind. What influenced me most was seeing the tears in her eyes as we spoke. For me, it was essential to reach the person inside the position. Perhaps this is why we need to see the humanity of God . . .

- What kind of patient are you to care for?
- What do you need from your doctor? If you're not getting it, what might you do?
- See the film *The Doctor* with William Hurt and recommend it to your doctor if you like it.

Why is it, God, that it is so hard for some of us to show our hearts, while others of us so desperately need to know with the heart? Help us to be patient enough with each other to find a common ground. Amen.

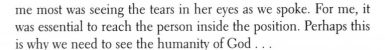

AS BEFORE when I've had cancer, my work as a counselor has kept me going. Perhaps it is the ability to focus on someone else's struggles and fears instead of my own. It has always been true for me that once I am in session with someone, I forget about myself. I am fascinated by their revelations and honored to be a part of their self-discovery. Whatever the situation, we are on a journey together, under God's protection and guidance. One of my current clients, Annie, is a particular favorite of mine. A Dutch survivor of Japanese camps during World War II, she is frail of body but strong of mind and spirit. At eighty-five, she still drives herself to church and cultural events, studies theology, paints, and visits shut-ins! One of her gifts to me is that, in every session, she asks—and insists on a truthful answer—"and so, Melody, how are you doing? Are you taking care of yourself?" Yes, we are all on a journey together . . . with the help of God.

· What kind of work do you do? Does your work help you to "keep going" right now? In what way? If not, what can be done about this?
· Is there a sense in which you feel "called by God" to your vocation? How?
· What "gifts" have you received from your clients or customers? Is there a mutuality in these relationships?

Let us leave room in our caring, O Lord, for the caring love of others. Amen.

THERE IS A GROUP of women in our church who love to go to movies. I am fortunate that they invited me to come along. Mostly, we attend foreign films—the kind with subtitles that don't usually make it to the "big screen," the ones that win awards at Cannes and Sundance Film Festivals. Great movies! Often, we stay for the discussion afterwards. If not, we go out and have our own discussion over a glass of wine or dessert. Truly food for mind, body, and soul! One wonderful side benefit from this group has been the development of a three-way friendship—"the terrific trio." Shirley, Carolyn, and I have become best buddies and celebrate birthdays and other occasions as a threesome.

· How do you feel about foreign films? Do you have a favorite?
· Can you recall being included in a group you wanted to be part of? (If not, what group might you start and invite others to?)

God, beyond the images that we make, be present to us in all that we see and hear. Let us find you in flickering lights and faithful friends, and nourish us all. Amen.

HELP! I know I had written more meditations a while ago when I went away with my friend Carol to the Cape—but I can't find them anywhere! They don't appear in any of my files or on any floppy disc I have. How could I let this happen?! I have never been a very organized or methodical person—I am too eclectic and prolific to keep it together for long—but this is inexcusable, even for me! I search frantically—and in vain—until I run out of possibilities. It is then that I sit myself down and try to "get a grip." Perhaps, I concluded, these were not ones that were ready to be shared and I need to make space for other ideas to emerge.

· How do you feel when you lose something important?
· What kind of person are you in terms of organization?
· Do you think there are higher reasons for things like this to happen?

God, you who continually bring order out of chaos, creation out of a void, life out of death: bring a sense of calm and purpose to our scattered souls, and allow us to see a clearer, deeper truth. Amen.

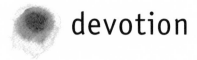 # devotion

IT IS MOTHER'S DAY and I am reminded of the passage where God declares to Israel the love that has existed even " . . . before I knit you in your mother's womb . . . ." This comforts me today as I am facing the beginning of a series of radiation treatments. It is also the first Mother's Day for me without my beloved mother. I miss her terribly but am glad she did not live to see me have to face this disease yet one more time.

How good it is to know that God, too, is my everlasting Mother! And that She is more than equal to the task of helping me in my fight against cancer. Her love will give me strength, hope, and courage.

I sang a solo in her (Her) honor in church this morning—and she (She) was smiling on me . . . I just know it!

· When, in your life, have you felt a "mother's love" when you most needed it? When not?
· Have there been others who have "mothered" you other than a parent?
· How do you feel about the image of God as "Mother"?

God, of all those in need of nurture and love, be as close to us this day as a mother's heart. Care for us, love us, hold us dear. Amen.

TUESDAY AGAIN. For some reason, I feel more down on Tuesdays—perhaps because it's really my "Monday," the start of my work week. And I don't know where I'm going to find the energy to see my clients. They need me for healing and yet, I need to rest and help myself to heal. As I'm slowly getting geared up for the day, the phone rings. It is my best friend from California, Shelley. She always cheers me with her sweet, loving spirit. I am able to laugh and cry with her—sometimes in the same breath—and there is such unshakable trust between us. When I first moved away, she promised me she'd come see me once a year—no matter where I lived—and she has done so every year for eight years now, from Iowa to Connecticut. When I had my last recurrence, she came and cooked for us even though she hates to and admits it is not her forte. I am strongly reminded of the story of Ruth and Naomi, as Shel is Jewish and I am Christian. We are still very much "sisters in spirit." My energy soars and I am ready to face the day, graced by the love of my precious friend.

- Have you had a friendship with someone outwardly very different from you? How has this enriched your life?
- Is there someone you've been wanting to get closer to? How could this happen?
- Write a letter to your "best friend"…

For friendship: offered, entered, promised, maintained, nurtured, and grown; we give you thanks, O God. Amen

SOMETIMES WE NEED to keep learning the same lesson over and over until we get it. Previous to my recurrence, I had plans in place to make a trip with friends to Guatemala—a combination education and mission trip. It was co-organized by two friends of mine from the Midwest: Diane, a high school counselor from South Dakota who had a second unpaid job placing children from one of the orphanages there for adoption (two of whom have become part of her own family), and Roxanne, my adopted "sister," a Native American student advisor at the University of Minnesota, who was leading a group of students to meet with indigenous peoples. I was especially excited to go because Roxanne's daughter Ronelle, whom I consider my "niece," was going as her thirteenth birthday present. Yet, as the time to go approached, I knew in my heart—and even more so in my body—that it would be best not to go. I continued to agonize and pray about it up until the last minute. Finally, I knew I had to make the call. Wonderfully, both of my friends were not only understanding but relieved. They, too, were worried about how physically demanding it might be for me in such primitive and, at times, dangerous conditions. Neither of them, however, wanted to make the decision for me. But as Roxanne said, "We love you and want what's best for you!" So must God feel about all our decisions—big and small.

- What lessons have you had to be taught over and over until you truly learned them?
- Are your mind and body ever in opposition to one another and how do you deal with this?
- Do you think God loves us enough to let us make our own decisions (and mistakes)? What might God be thinking about some of the decisions you're facing right now?

Give us the courage and the wisdom to live in the reality of our limitations, God, but never to give in to the limitation of your reality. Let us live in truthful hope. Amen.

ONE OF THE REASONS I like my oncologist is her nurse, Bonnie. From our first meeting, I knew I'd found a kindred spirit. Not only is she a competent, experienced professional, but she is a warm, funny, spontaneous, quirky soul. Never did she fail to make me laugh (which was a real trick sometimes, given how upset, tired, anxious, or fearful I could get). More importantly, I felt she always saw me as a unique individual, worthy of special attention, no matter what. For my IV treatments, she found me a private space with a couch and a phone—as if I were the only patient she had to cater to. This must be the way God sees each one of us—as a beloved, only child!

· Do you have a "Bonnie" in your life? Tell her/him how she/he helps you (if you haven't already).
· During this illness, can you recall humor and laughter being a part of the experience? In what way? If not, why not?
· Have you ever felt really "special"—like an "only child"? What was this like for you?

Thank you, God, for the attentive joy that allows us to appreciate the blessings of life, even as we work to enrich and protect it. For those who care for us and laugh with us, we are grateful. Amen.

UPON FIRST RECEIVING the diagnosis of recurrence, Richard and I are both stunned and saddened. I spend the night crying and fretting in his arms—he, too, in a "blue funk." What would we do without each other to help bear this bad news? The next day, though, we are already phoning to set up an appointment for a second opinion. As soon as we're able to get a time and gather all my medical records, we're off to Boston. Dana Farber Women's Clinic is an ultramodern state-of-the art facility near Boston University. It is a hands-on kind of place with greeters at every station, pleasant, helpful, and reassuring. The doctor herself, Karen Craig, is a pretty, friendly woman who talks and shares openly with us. After examining me, she states she is not at all sure it is a recurrence—but is "curious"—so she is ordering yet more tests to determine what it is (even though, later, it turns out to be cancer again). Instead of feeling "terminally unique," I feel hope for the first time in at least a week. This doctor, like the Divine Physician, has seen my worst possible fear and put it in a positive light. There is always Hope . . .

· Can you recall your first response to the diagnosis of "cancer"?
· Who was there for you during that time and in what way?
· Is there someone like Dr. Craig who has given you hope when you sorely needed it? Do they realize this?

Give us the perseverance to seek more information, the patience to wait for it to come, and the perspective to deal with whatever reality we find. In other words, give us faith. Amen.

MY DEAR FRIEND Shelley comes to visit. She has moved up her trip this year because she is worried about me. As always, the time is too short but we make the most of it. We do this by simply focusing on "being" rather than doing. Shel is one of those rare friends with whom I can do this. There is a gentle intensity to our friendship that allows us to shut out everything else. Today, we decide to hang out at the house. Shelley wants to help me so she cleans my refrigerator—something that badly needs doing!—while I plant flowers. We check in with one another but are happy just to be quietly in the same space. Afterwards, we sip lemonade and sit in the hammock together. It is a true blessing to be so at home with another person. Friends are God in human form, I decide.

· Have you had a best friend like Shelley? Where is that person in your life right now?
· Is there anyone you feel so completely "at home with" as this? What makes this possible?
· Write a letter or poem to this friend, telling him or her how you feel. (Be sure to mention God somewhere in it.)

Help us, God, to be comfortable enough with others that we can neither enter their "space" nor have them encroach upon ours; that we can simply be in the same place together. Amen.

THERE IS A COUPLE in our church that Richard and I say remind us of ourselves—the selves we believe we will be at their age. Ed and Edith are in their eighties, a beautiful, gracious Scandinavian pair who just celebrated their sixtieth anniversary. It was a quiet celebration as they are both in poor health but rich in spirit and love for one another. They are each caregivers to the other. She finishes his sentences, as he is quite deaf, and laughs at his jokes and stories, many of which she has heard before. He drives her around even though he really can't see all that well, and he believes her to be the loveliest woman in the world. Soon, they are moving to a retirement home and we are buying their dining room set. We hope it brings with it some of their loving and generous relationship that we can soak up and share with one another.

· Who do you think you'll be like as you age?
· How does your coupleness express itself?
· Is love "blind"? What about God's love?

Help us to see each other through the eyes of love and Love. Let our experiences of one another paint our images of beauty, and let your blessing of life fill us with renewing joy. Amen.

6

compassion

I HAVE BEEN ORPHANED TWICE. At age three, I was adopted after living the first three years of my life in a foster home. My adoptive parents were loving and close, never making me feel anything less than their beloved, chosen daughter. My father died nine years ago at age ninety-one and my mother this spring at age seventy-five. So, once again, I am an orphan—this time at age fifty-one! Thankfully, my mother's three sisters—Thelma, Verda, and Arline—have kept in contact with me since her death. It is as if they made a promise to not leave me "motherless." Their letters and phone calls always lift me up and remind me that I am loved by family. Each of them, like my mother, is a woman of deep faith, having had this tested in many ways over the years. They remember my mother to me in their words and their mannerisms. I am so very grateful to God that I have my "aunties" no matter how old I become!

· Have you ever felt "orphaned" (in the sense of abandoned or alone)?
· Do you have aunties (or uncles) or other folks like them in your life? Pick one and write a letter, telling that person how much they have meant to you (feel free to send it or not).
· What do you think of when you hear or read the phrase "woman (or man) of faith"? Do you see yourself at all in this description?

Remember your promises, God, to never leave us. We've been left enough as it is. Be with us. Amen.

I HAD A VERY POSITIVE EXPERIENCE today with the hospital staff assisting me in getting a CAT Scan. (So unlike my first experience in radiation!) From the time the technician came to get me in the waiting room, he was calm and gentle in his tone, his words, and his movements, all of which helped me to be as well. There was an attentiveness to detail and comfort (was I cold?) and a reassuring hand on my shoulder. The nurse who came to flush and connect my port was also a caring person, the sort who put me immediately at ease. When she led me to the other room, she held me by the hand, unselfconsciously, and it felt OK to be tended to like a child.

· Have you had corrective emotional experiences in your treatment?
· How important is touching to you and how does it affect you?
· In what ways does this reflect God's love for God's children?

Let the care we receive be truly caring, O God. Work through those with skill, that they may touch us with healing compassion as well. Amen.

WE CHURCH PEOPLE are often at our best when the need becomes the greatest. It is when someone is in crisis or there is a death in the family that we rise to the occasion. Perhaps it is because, in these instances, what is needed is clear and concrete—the four C's of congregational life: compassion, cards, calls, and casseroles! My illness was no exception. In fact, perhaps because I am the pastor's wife, I received more than my share of the above. Hardly a day passed that I did not have tangible proof that I was being thought of and prayed for. Many things touched me—too numerous to mention here—but two especially stand out. A new friend, Bainie, sent a lovely card in which she had enclosed a gold chain with a graceful butterfly on it. "Grace-full" is the word for it. The attached note said that this had been worn by both her mother and herself during difficult periods in their lives, and that she wanted me to have it as long as I needed it. Whenever I wear this, I feel a special connection to her and to the God of new life symbolized by the butterfly.

Then, another new friend, Angie, brought me a stuffed animal, showing me not only that she cared but that she really listened to me. Once, during a bell choir rehearsal, I remarked that my lack of rhythm made me feel like "a hippopotamus in a tutu" (à la *Fantasia*). Well, guess what Angie found? I keep my stuffed hippo on the sofa in my counseling office to remind myself that I am rhythmically challenged and therefore not perfect, but that, even so, I am kind of appealing in a cute and silly sort of way. This helps me to remember to lighten up on myself and others.

- Have there been "church people" (people from your faith community) who have helped you? In what ways?
- What is your relationship to the wife/husband (or significant other) of your spiritual leader? Do the members of your faith community practice the four C's? What else?
- Are there creatures from the natural realm—animals—with which you identify? Draw a picture of yourself as that creature …

We are all hippopotami, we are all butterflies: help us to love each, in all of us, and in ourselves. Amen.

AS A PASTOR'S SPOUSE, I've learned the importance of making friends outside our church. When I move to a new town, I start by contacting people in my field for potential "friendships." That is how I met my new friend Valerie. Val is a short, cute, energetic and passionate extrovert who lives life to its fullest. We quickly graduated from talking over coffee to talking and walking our dogs together once a week, rain or shine. With my recurrence, however, the doctor didn't want me to walk my dog Sam as he might pull or twist me, reinjuring my fragile hip. Val decided we could still walk as long as she handled both dogs and I just took care of myself. That was quite a challenge for my diminutive but determined friend—but she wanted to do it for me and so we did. While we walked—more slowly than usual—she kept an eye out so the dogs wouldn't bump or jostle me. I felt so cared for and recalled Jesus speaking tenderly of caring for His sheep . . .

· How do you go about "making friends"?
· Have you ever had a friend, like Val, who has really "put herself out" for you? In what way?
· Can you relate to the parable of the Good Shepherd? How do you experience God's compassion and care?

God of loving opportunity, thank you for the many ways you make it possible for us to care about each other, and for the people who walk in those ways. Amen.

ONE OF MY CURRENT favorite songs by John Astin is entitled "Love, Serve, and Remember." It has a lovely, lilting chorus that goes "Why have we come to earth? Why have we taken birth? . . . To love, serve, and remember . . . " I always want to end the song by shouting "Amen!" but that is not how it was written. In my understanding, the word "Amen" means "so be it." For me, saying this is a way to move myself from belief to action. I believe I have this disease so I can be reminded of the purpose of my life on this earth: to love, serve, and remember. None of these three is whole without the others; together, they form the essence of life in the Spirit.

- Do you ever ask yourself the questions as posed in this song? Do any answers come to you?
- Have you ever wanted to shout "Amen!" out loud? Did you? How did it feel?
- What do you think of this notion of "a purpose to this disease"? What might yours be?

Let me remember you, God; let me love you, God; let me serve you, God. Amen. Amen. Amen.

LIKE MANY WOMEN (and some men), I've been keeping a diary off and on since adolescence. As an adult, I've gone through periods of keeping a journal—mostly in times of transition and crisis, however. A few years ago, I even took a journal writing workshop focused on spirituality. All of this has taught me that the most important thing about journaling is to do it! The next most important is to remember it's just for me. This book of meditations started as that—a personal account. Then, about midway through my treatment—journaling each day—I knew I was writing this also for others like myself. I can remember the time and place: it was during the quiet, morning meditation time on the loveseat in my office. The clock was ticking steadily, the light streaming softly. I was all alone with God and my thoughts. And suddenly, I knew I had to do this. Naturally, the next thought was "Why me? Who am I to think I have something important or original to say to others?" Yadayadayada . . . You get the idea. Despite these nagging and irritating doubts, here I am, pen in hand, and glad of it! Whatever comes of this is a gift from God . . .

· Have you ever kept a journal or a diary? When? How was this for you?
· If you're able, dig out your journal and spend some time rereading it. Reflect on the person you meet in its pages.
· Do you feel you might have something worthwhile to share with others? (Dare to put it down right here and now!).

Grant us the grace to be willing to share the insights and the experiences and the wisdom of our lives, so that we may be fulfilled by the telling, and others enriched by the hearing. Amen.

WITH THIS RECURRENCE and subsequent chemotherapy, I have lost not only my appetite but quite a lot of weight as well. Now, ordinarily, like most women, I wouldn't mind this—but I am really quite thin and could use some extra weight to keep up my strength. As a result, everyone around me is now on a mission to put some pounds back on Melody. This takes the form of tempting me with goodies, taking me out to eat, and frequent, loving reminders to "clear your plate!" Several of the folks at church have taken to bringing tasty, homemade dishes to my doorstep. This is such a wonderful ministry to both me and my family. I don't really have the energy to plan meals and Richard, though an excellent and creative cook, is too scattered to focus on much else right now. Two couples have been especially generous to us. Ron and Petie, newlyweds who by all rights could be tuned in only to each other, have brought several of their own favorite dishes to share with us. David and Margaret have not only prepared extra barbeque dinners for us but have gone out and purchased liquid protein supplements for me to drink. It is a standing joke that, when I see David, the mantra has become, "Eat, eat, eat . . ."

· Have you struggled with weight issues during your illness?
· What is it like for you to be truly fed, nurtured in a physical way, by someone else?
· Write a bit about the spiritual significance of being fed by another.

Bread of Life, nourish us. Water of Life, refresh us. Source of Life, restore us, by your grace. Amen.

FOOD, TO ME, is one of life's greatest pleasures. Perhaps some of this stems from my Chinese background as well as growing up in a restaurant family. Food was definitely love in our household! Which is why I was so touched today by the offer made at church to bring us dinner this evening. Doris, a lively and lovely woman my mother's age, said she was making homemade macaroni and cheese—"my daughter's favorite"—and would be happy to make an extra one for us. Little did she know how much I'd been missing my mom's home cooking (and TLC). When she arrived with the dish, steaming, fragrant, and very "cheesy," I wanted to cry and hug it to my chest. Instead, I ate way too many helpings and had a full but contented tummy. Truly "comfort food."

· What is your relationship to food? Friend or foe? What has it meant to you?
· Recall the last time you got "fed" by someone and really "took it in" . . .

· Name your "comfort food(s)." Be sure to have at least one of these a week, beginning this week.

Food for thought; food for the soul; food: for feeding us, we give you thanks, O God. Amen.

It is not always true that good things come in small packages. Today, we received a most wonderful, extremely large, gift. It wasn't wrapped—but that would have been quite a challenge. A very generous couple from our church, Dick and Angela Maine, gave us their Ford Explorer! They were purchasing a new vehicle for themselves and decided, rather than trade it in or sell it, to give it to us. They were concerned that our aging vehicles wouldn't make it through another New England winter (and they may well have been right about this). We were overwhelmed by their gesture and overjoyed to get this vehicle. Their attitude was "don't mention it—we're just glad we can do it and it works for you." Talk about good stewards of the resources God has given them!

· What is the most unexpected gift you've received during this illness? (Make it something physical and concrete.)
· Has anyone ever overwhelmed you with generosity? How did you react? Write a thank you note to that person.
· Do you see yourself as a "good steward" of the resources God has given you?

Generosity amazes us, O God. Help us to be more generous, so that it becomes more frequent, and less unusual. Amen.

LIKE MANY PEOPLE of my generation, I struggle with the unanswerable, timeless questions more than I probably need to. We were raised and trained to be socially conscious, involved, relevant, and politically correct. Kind of a burden sometimes. And yet, as they say, it is our "cross to bear," isn't it? Therefore, when someone like me gets cancer, it's not simply a matter of "a personal problem"; rather, it's seen as a problem that needs to be addressed on a communal and societal level. We are none of us isolated entities. What can be done about it is not even as important as the context in which we consider it—our frame of reference, our motivations. For me, this passage from Micah 6:8 has become my own answer to what I expect of myself based on what God—not self or others—expects from me. "He has told you, O mortal, what is good; and what does [God] require of you but to do justice, and to love kindness, and to walk humbly with your God."

- What was the "ethos" of the time in which you were raised? How has this affected the kind of person you have become?
- Any reflections on the Micah 6:8 passage? Does it stir you in any way?
- Do you have a favorite passage or writing that inspires and guides your life? Why is this?

We seek the strength, O God, to insist on the healing of the cancers of injustice and mercilessness and arrogance that keep your people from being fully whole. Even as we long for health in our own bodies, so do we pray for that day when the decisions of "the people" will be made with people at heart. Help us to love all of us, as do you. Amen.

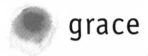

grace

ONE OF MY HOSPICE PATIENTS gave me a lovely gift today. Now, I know counselors aren't supposed to accept gifts from clients, but I've decided it's ridiculous and perhaps even cruel to refuse small gifts from one who is dying. Having been a patient myself, I recognize how very important it is to be able to give as well as receive as long as one is able. Anyway, this gift really didn't amount to much materially. My client is a wonderful flower gardener—everything grows under her thumb—and her specialty is showy spring flowers. With her failing energy, she dug up hundreds of bulbs, of which she gave me several dozen to plant in the fall in my fledgling garden. It is comforting to us both to be cultivating the same flowers—from one garden and one spirit to another . . .

· Is it hard for you to let others "give" to you right now?
· Can you think of ways in which you might "give" to those around you?
· Be aware—today—of the "gifts" given and received in your life.

Give us the gracious wisdom it takes to accept gifts, O God, because we know that our day will be filled with them. Amen.

MY BROTHER DAN is a youth minister in a Cornerstone Christian Fellowship. It is a congregation outwardly very different from ours in New England. Whereas our church members tend to be more established and prosperous, Dan's tend to be folks who are marginal and struggling. Yet, they have a deep joy and richness of spirit that is infectious. Perhaps because they have had to deal with so much hard reality, they are more openly grateful and humble. When I last worshipped with them, I felt especially taken in by them, as "one of the family." It was a delight to be in worship and play. I felt accepted and free "just as I am . . ." Praise God!

· To what kind of congregation do you belong?
· Have you been exposed to other styles of worship?
· How do you think God might feel about all this?

Accept us as we are, O God, and give to us the wisdom and the grace to realize and embrace that acceptance. Let us love ourselves, as you have loved us. Amen.

WHILE SEATED in a hallway full of patients waiting to be called into an examining room so they can wait to be seen, I am greeted warmly by a very attractive African American woman in street clothes. She introduces herself to me as Robin, one of the support staff in the Oncology Department. She recognizes me by name, which surprises me. Sitting in this hallway, one really begins to feel like a "nonentity." I perk up as she connects me with my husband's church. It seems she is taking her daughter there to look at our preschool program. I share my opinion of its excellence and we chat for a few minutes. As she leaves, I find myself renewed for having been "seen"—not as a patient but as a person beyond the one waiting in a blue hospital gown. Just so, God sees each one of us as special people, with something valuable to contribute.

· Can you recall a time when you were "recognized" unexpectedly by someone? How did this feel?
· How about the experience of feeling like a "nonentity"?
· Are there places in your life where you can escape being a "patient" and just be a "person"?

Thank you, God, for the connections that enable us to see another and to be seen, and to know that in our differences we are one. Amen.

BEING A PASTOR'S FAMILY, we are blessed with so many friends in our congregation. This one is especially rich for us in that they have welcomed us from the beginning as "one of them." As a result, we continually have many invitations to be among them. Right now, being in treatment, this feels incredibly affirming and "normalizing." Tonight, we spent an evening filled with music, good food, and much laughter. I feel filled up with love and life! It is particularly poignant in that no one ever mentioned my cancer. For this one evening, I was just one of the gang—God's "Little Rascals"!

· In what places do you feel most welcomed in your life?
· Are there ever times where you "forget" you have cancer (even for a little while)?
· Ask people close to you not to bring "it" up just for a day (and remember: you can't either!) ...

Remind us, dear God, that we are all your children, created in your image to love you . . . and one another. Amen.

THERE ARE TIMES in my life when I am absolutely overwhelmed by the goodness of people. Today was one of those times. I knew when I came home for a visit that I wanted to see some dear friends who live in the Midwest. I also knew I wasn't ready to visit a city where we'd experienced so much pain. In our nearly eight-year ministry there, we managed to serve in an extremely dysfunctional church, a true "clergy-killing" congregation. (We certainly didn't thrive there—we survived!) So, I had to ask my friends to make the trek up to see me instead. Two friends, Cyndi and Frank, not only traveled six hours from home but stopped to pick up another friend, Gloria, on the way—a total of nine hours driving! When I tried to thank them, they could only say, "We are glad to do it—we all need to see our friends." Such generosity not only touches me but also reminds me that God is so gracious to us!

· When have you been overwhelmed by the goodness of others?
· Are there places in your life where you cannot go?
· How has God's graciousness been shown to you?

Where the bonds of love and care are strong, we pray that we have the chance to reach out, and to be reached. Where there are hurts and resentments in our path, may your love, O God, yet find a way. Amen.

ONE OF OUR FAVORITE older couples in the church is Dave and June Berg. They are one of those couples whose relationship seems to have blossomed even more since retirement. They are truly enjoying life and each other to the fullest—no jobs or children to worry about on a daily basis (I hope fervently to get to this point someday with my own dear husband). Today, Dave and June have invited us to go to a concert at Tanglewood with them.

It is a Saturday morning rehearsal of the Boston Pops conducted by Seizi Ozawa—someone I have only dreamed of seeing in person. After a delicious brunch on the lawn, prepared by June, we take our seats in the outdoor amphitheater—only a few rows behind the orchestra. It is breathtaking! As the music wafts over us, some of it seeps into my sore bones and aching soul and it lifts me up, soothing pain and fear. How can life possibly end when there is so much music yet to be heard? . . .

- Do you have a "favorite couple" in your life? Why are they special to you?
- Is there something, like the Tanglewood concert (or Seiji Ozawa, to be exact!), that you long to attend? How might this happen for you?
- What, as music does for me, lifts you up beyond the present reality of your illness?

Sing, choirs of angels: sing in . . . exaltation, joy, hope, peace, healing, love, friendship . . . sing in our hearts. Amen.

THIS MORNING, I attended a memorial service for a hospice client. It was held in a lovely large Congregational church in downtown Hartford and the church was packed. Almost late—as usual—I slipped into a pew in the back as quietly as possible. It is strange, being a counselor, because we become so very close to people at extremely sensitive times—and yet, we are also "outsiders." Still, I felt moved by the words—and the silences—in the service. Greeting the family afterwards, I felt sadness for their loss and also for mine, as I would probably not see them again. Driving home, tears flowing, I thought that this must be how my healers felt towards me—and especially how the Divine Healer feels towards each of us. When we are suffering and in pain, God's presence can be quite palpable—almost like another heart beating in rhythm along with ours. Yet, there is also a way in which we are honored enough by God that we are enabled to go on living on our own. That is how much God loves us!

· Have you ever felt like an "outsider" in a gathering of folks you know intimately? What was this like for you?
· Try to get in touch with the "heart of God" in just a small way. How might God feel when you are ill or hurting?
· Do you think there are people who might feel this way about you? Name them and let yourself be with them in spirit . . .

Let us be open to being cared for, enriched, ministered to, loved. Let us not become so filled by what we ought to do that we do not receive what we are offered. Amen.

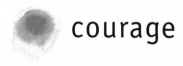 # courage

8

I STARTED radiation treatments today. This was my first experience, though I've had chemotherapy twice before, and I didn't know just what to expect. The previous day I'd been told by the orthopedist that my bones were strong enough to withstand radiation (I guess good news is relative!). The technicians were in a hurry, didn't take time to explain the procedures, and were, in general, rather impersonal. Combined with my anxiety and "need to know," this did not sit well with me. So, instead of holding it in, in an effort to be the "good patient," I shared my distress and frustration with them. I was sorry I'd done so at first, because it made things rather awkward and tense between us (not at all what either one of us wanted or needed). Initially taken aback and responding defensively, they later called to apologize and to set up a meeting for me with the head nurse and oncology social worker. I believe all of this will help to bridge the gap between us and get us off to a better start.

- Recall your first day of treatment. What was it like? How were you treated? How did you relate to others?
- Is there someone in your life to whom you need to "speak the truth in love"? Feel free to write here what you would like to say …
- Is there a "truth" you need to share with God alone? (Again, feel free to do so here …)

Help us learn how to truly speak the truth in love, O God of both. And, having learned how, help us to do so. Amen.

THE FIRST DAY of the second week of radiation therapy. (Why am I reminded of a prisoner in a cell, marking days on the wall?) At any rate, it was rather hard to gear myself up for beginning again, after a weekend off, and a very nice weekend at that. As I reluctantly got into the car to head for the hospital, the phrase "All you have to do is show up . . ." popped into my head, followed by ". . . and I'll take care of the rest." Now, I wondered, had I gotten to the point where I was delusional? Hearing voices? Being a psychotherapist is not always easy—we analyze ourselves worst of all. But I don't think it was anything of the sort. I believe it was God letting me know—in a way I could "hear"—that all I really needed to do was to take the next step . . . and that Someone else would take if from there.

- Reflect on the times in this experience when you have felt like a prisoner marking off the days . . .
- Picture yourself being released from the cell that holds you. What would this be like?
- Have you ever "heard voices"? How about the voice of God?

Grant us the courage to show up, God. Help us to take the steps to get through the morning, the noon, the evening, and the night and all the moments along the way. Keep us from disappearing from our own lives. Amen.

SOME OCCASIONS ARE MADE for sharing and celebration. This was one of them. Today was the last official day of radiation therapy for me. Oh, I'll have lots of tests and follow-up appointments but no more "zapping"—at least for now. It was a heady and liberating feeling to leave the hospital the last time, hugged and wished well by all my technicians and even given a graduation "diploma."

Then, there was a temporary letdown—back to life as usual—but not for long! In the evening, a guitarist friend, John, and I sang at the local Relay for Life, a national event sponsored by the American Cancer Society. It was a wonderful event with walkers, joggers, speakers, and a luminary ceremony honoring those who have died and those who are living with cancer. So many names on bags of sand, lit with candles in a formation that spelled out "HOPE." Indeed! In introducing myself, I shared that I, too, am a cancer survivor and I was cheered. Nothing in my life could make me feel more of a champion than that moment. Buoyed by the best wishes of those gathered, hundreds of strangers, save a few, I sang and John played like we'd never done in all our rehearsals. Truly the Spirit was with us!

· What have been your experiences of "graduations" of your own?
· Imagine yourself being "cheered" as a cancer survivor....What might this be like?
· Define "champion" and try this on to see if it fits at all for you.

Lift our spirits, God, with words of hope and accomplishment and respect. Let us realize and accept how very wonderful we are. Amen.

I'M INVITED to a meeting of hospice social workers—one of our rare and enjoyable social gatherings outside of work. Due to my radiation and flagging energy, I have not seen them all summer since I haven't gone to any staff meetings. They, however, have been wonderful in keeping in touch via notes and phone messages. On the way, driven by my dear, protective husband (who doesn't want me to get too tired), I experience a combination of excitement and apprehension. Why the latter? I wonder. Reflecting, I realize I will be glad to see them all again but worry that they'll relate to me as sick and dying (an occupational hazard?). Upon arriving, I am greeted enthusiastically by my colleagues who treat me as they always did—as one of them. Even though I have only been on staff for less than six months, I have been accepted from the beginning. We are, after all, comrades in the same struggle, coping with fear, pain, loss, and grief—all aspects of this brief span we call life. I recognize that, in me, they see life only because, in You, I have Life!

- Are there people who have kept in touch with you during your illness in unexpected and pleasing ways? Name them and say a prayer of thanksgiving for their presence in your life.
- Do you ever get your feelings all "mixed up"—like mine of excitement and apprehension—and, if so, what helps you to untangle them?
- Write a statement expressing your view on being ill rather than being the illness. Put this by your mirror and read it (at least) each morning and evening …

Help us hold on to the truth that we are not our disease. We are the gifts and the talents and the interests and the loves that have always connected us to others. We are health, not illness. Amen.

WHILE RICHARD WAS A CANDIDATE for his current position, the church held a couple of receptions to introduce us to members of the congregation. One of the first persons we met was Terry, a bubbly, bright woman our age who told us she was relieved to learn we had been divorced, as she was. Soon after coming here, we discovered yet another point of commonality: Terry developed cancer. Hers is a particularly difficult kind, as it has spread and is especially resistant to treatment. Yet, Terry is tough and willing to try any—and every—thing possible. She has been on rigorous chemotherapy longer than anyone I know without a break—but with little results. She has lost her hair but not her hope. She lives alone, continues to work when she can, stays in touch with friends and family, and "keeps the faith." Today, she invited me to go with her to a faith healer she has been seeing. I'm not sure how I felt about this faith healer, a well-meaning but unusual woman who uses both touch and intuition to effect healing. I am sure how I feel about Terry: a mix of fondness, admiration, concern, and sisterhood. We are women warriors, side by side in battle, fighting the good fight with all our might . . .

· Is there someone you know who is going through cancer at the same time as you? What is your connection with that person like?
· Would you like to be closer? How might this happen?
· Describe (or write a poem or draw a picture of) what a "woman warrior" is like …

We are not resentful, O God, for the limits cancer has placed upon our lives; we are grateful for the new people and meanings you have brought us that we might otherwise have missed. Amen.

IN EVERY STAGE of dealing with cancer, it has helped me tremendously to have other people who have "been there." This time around, one of them has been Penny, a lovely lady from church. Penny is one of those women who one can tell was beautiful when young, and who has become even more so with age, in a delicate, soft way. She is an artist who struggles with painful arthritis, and she now has had to undergo a series of radiation treatments for breast cancer. I know these have made her very tired and yet, every time I see her, she inquires about my progress in a most tender manner. I can feel her exhaustion, but even more, I feel her reaching out to me to give me encouragement. It is as if she is communicating "You'll get through this—we both will." And I believe her because she's been there.

- Are there people who have "been there" in your life? What role do they play for you?
- Do you think older people can be "beautiful"? How so?
- What do you imagine you'll look like when you're "old" (in words or a picture …?

Remind us that we need not go through our trials alone, O God: that you send us messenger angels at every turn to show us the way. Amen.

ON OUR WAY to Boston where I have a doctor's appointment for a second opinion, we stop to see Art and Millie Tucker, members of our congregation. Millie has been battling breast cancer for a few years and is in the end stages of this all-too-common disease. She now has hospice and only sees close family and friends for short periods. Art is her primary caregiver and he is tirelessly devoted to her care. They have a solid, strong bond that has spanned five decades. Both of them are tiny, wiry, active, and intelligent— quiet doers and stewards—backbones of our church and community. New Englanders in the best sense. Today, though, they both look tired, tense, and sad. Fighting this disease is taking a toll on them. It is obvious how much energy this has all taken and how little is left at this point. Close to tears on parting, they remark how kind it was of us to take our time to stop and be with them. I am struck by the irony of this because, to me, it is their time that is limited and so very precious—not ours.

· How do you feel when you know "the end is near" for you or someone else you care about?
· Are you able to be sensitive to yourself or others when the need is to close down or withdraw?
· Where are you from? Can you see how your roots or heritage affect the way you cope with the disease?

Grant us the grace, O God, to meet graciousness halfway. Amen.

IT IS TRUE that cancer, like many major illnesses, is a leveler, a common denominator among people who live with it. Like it or not, we have much in common with one another—too much. A church member, Lois, was recently diagnosed with "inoperable lung cancer." In her eighties, she has the energy of someone half her age. Her life is rich with friends, family, and activities. She is, in no way, ready to depart this world. On Sunday mornings, during our joys and concerns, she asks for prayers for herself—"and for Melody, too."

· What do people living with cancer have in common?
· Are you ready to depart this world?
· Have you had someone ask for prayers for you?

Hear our prayers, O God, for ourselves, and for all those who share our fears and our hopes, our challenges and our triumphs. Let the voices of our spirits rise in chorus to Thee. Amen.

TODAY, I GAVE my yearly sermon—the one I give when Richard is off on Continuing Education. He has always been a supportive mentor to me; it is I who compare myself to him and decline to preach when he is present. (Maybe I'll get over this; I hope so.) This time, I actually enjoyed giving today's sermon. It was one of those that almost preached itself. The topic was one very close to my heart—and I believe, to the heart of God—that of healing prayer. I emphasized the crucial first step of finding inner peace—through prayer—before healing, whether physical, emotional, or spiritual, can occur. Folks were wonderfully receptive and it felt like a dialogue between us.

· Have you ever "preached" or taught to a group? How was it?
· In what way do you undermine your own confidence and effectiveness?
· What topic is on your heart that you might like to share with others?

Help us find the words to give expression to our faith, our God. Grant us the courage to speak and the humility to listen. Be the ever-present listening voice in all our dialogues of hope. Amen.

CANCER "MAKES STRANGE BEDFELLOWS," to borrow a phrase. My dear friend Gloria from Sioux City was diagnosed with "aggressive breast cancer" about six months ago. Since then, she has been undergoing various forms of chemotherapy and radiation with all the accompanying debilitating side effects. We have been in close contact by e-mail and, when I was in the Twin Cities, she came up to see me. Both of us were anxious to see one another with our own eyes—each to check out how the other was really doing. It was a bittersweet pleasure to be with her because her prognosis is not very optimistic, though she has a strong, fighting spirit. We were able to laugh and cry a bit together, share cancer "war stories," and be one another's mirrors. Sometimes it is easier to love and accept in someone else what it is difficult to accept in oneself.

· Is there someone close to you with whom you have cancer in common?
· What is it like to be with someone else going through a similar cancer experience?
· Write a prayer for this person.

Be present, O God, in the ones like us: those who struggle and fear, those who ennoble and hope, those who "know." Amen.

I HAVE YET ANOTHER recurrence of cancer. It has been very discouraging and frightening to me, as it seems to be both speeding up and spreading in the last few years. Furthermore, after numerous tests and consultations, I have begun on a course of chemotherapy, which will continue until the cancer is, hopefully, once again in remission. My doctor assures me that we have quite a few options left to us and reminds me that I have been very receptive to chemotherapy in the past. Both these thoughts help me to feel somewhat less anxious.

Before I had my first treatment today, I had to have some X-rays done. The two technicians were both young, pretty women, upbeat, and sensitive with me. One even put her hands together in an attitude of prayer and nodded at me as I left. It was the woman technician who did not even enter the room but worked on the machines next to us who had the most impact on me, however. While I was lying on the table, I could hear her humming, then softly singing songs in Spanish. I was too far away to hear the words distinctly, but by the sounds, I guessed she was singing praise songs. She was the one who walked me out to the waiting room and, on an impulse, I asked if she had a moment. She seemed surprised but quickly sat down and gave me her full attention. I inquired about her songs and she admitted that she had been praising God in Spanish. When I shared that I do the same in English, she relaxed and opened up with me. A strong Hispanic Catholic, she is active in her church and also leads spiritual retreats. She was pleased to learn that I do some of the same things in my church and that I will be entering into a program of Spiritual Direction at a seminary sponsored by her diocese. It was a close and warm few minutes we spent together. As I got up to leave, she grabbed my hand and said, "Praise God!" to which I replied, without thinking, "in all circumstances!" That had to come from the Holy Spirit because it wasn't me . . .

- Do you ever have the feeling that this cancer just won't let you go? How does this affect you?
- Can you sense the presence of God in your medical team? Is there a difference for you?
- Have you experienced an instance when you felt the words that came out of your mouth were from Someone else? What was this like for you?

You know, O God, that the cancer within is an uninvited and unwelcome intruder, doing its ill even as we work and pray against it. We ask that you be both invited and welcome in our hearts, spirits, minds, and bodies, and that you do us good at every turn. Gracias a Dios. Amen.

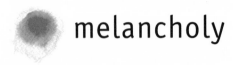

melancholy

9

WHEN ONE PERSON in a family is in pain or distress, all are affected. Naturally, we know this but we sometimes forget when we're in the middle of a difficult or frightening situation like a recurrence of cancer. This afternoon, I was driving Josh to an appointment after school. On our way there, I realized I'd left the directions at home—in a hurry, as usual. So I pulled up to a local gas station to look up the address. I stayed behind the wheel expecting Josh to go in, as I was in some physical discomfort. When he protested, I crabbily got out, slamming the car door. When I returned, I found him in tears. As we talked, he shared how tired he was of my being sick and how scared he was that I might not get well. My first reaction was to feel twinges of shame and guilt—how could I not know this? But these feelings quickly gave way to ones of love and gratitude. Thank you, God, for bringing conflict so we could get to clarity and compassion for one another!

- When you lose your way, where do you seek direction?
- Who in your life are you likely to take for granted during this time?
- How can you bring the "hard feelings" out in the open so you can each be there for one another?

We pray for the wisdom, O God, to discern the feelings and motivations behinds our actions and our words. Amen.

ANOTHER BEAUTIFUL SPRING DAY! A day of sunshine and showers both. I couldn't find my son, Josh, anywhere after dinner. I searched everywhere and finally found him sitting in the living room with the lights off, in the dark, alone. "Why didn't you answer me?" I crossly inquired. He didn't reply but just looked sad. So, instead of asking more, I simply sat beside him, sensing no need for words, just for presence. How often many of us yearn for just that! A quiet, loving, supportive presence. And God, Presence, is always there—if we can allow ourselves to be quiet enough to receive . . .

· Is being "quiet" hard for you? Do you know why this is?

· "Just do it!" and see what happens. (Afterward, write or draw your feelings here ...)

Shhhh. Amen.

IF I WERE to give one word to describe my work with hospice patients, it would be "bittersweet." Such a mixture of emotions all blended together at the end! Today was one of those days full of so many feelings that I know I will not ever forget. I had been working with the Cottos, a close and loving Puerto Rican couple. They had just celebrated their twenty-fifth wedding anniversary, still like newlyweds, when the wife was diagnosed with inoperable cancer. She was failing fast and had been in some discomfort, though not pain, and had a great deal of anxiety. Entering her room today, I knew something was different. There was a stillness and a peace in the air. When she opened her eyes, she smiled and asked me in Spanish if I saw the angels. I said no, but that I believed they were there. Her face was radiant and beautiful like a young girl's. Her husband joined us at her bedside with his guitar and sang love songs to her. All of us were in tears but full of joy as well. Never has love been as palpable—nor as holy—as in that room.

· Have you ever been in touch with the "bittersweet" in your life? What was "bitter"? What was "sweet"?

· Is there anyone in your life that you have ever felt as close to as with this couple? Do they realize this as well? Write about this relationship here …

· Do you believe in angels? Have you had any personal experiences with them?

Keep our eyes open, God, for your messengers and their music. Let us not miss the next visit of los angeles. Amen.

IN MY LIVING with cancer, I have been blessed by having friends in the same situation. We are comrades in spirit and struggle. One of those closest to me is Vivian, a friend from church who has lived with chronic health problems for twenty-five years, as long as she's been married to John. Lately, she seems to be losing the battle to cancer diagnosed less than a year ago. It is now in her liver and the doctor says there is nothing more he can do. Recently, she was accepted into an experimental program at Georgetown University Hospital—her "last hope." When we spoke after her first treatment, a rigorous mega-chemo isolation regime, she was exhausted and tearful. At one point, she asked me, "Mel, is it time for me to give up?"

- Are there fellow comrades in your struggle with cancer?
- How might you feel if your doctor told you what Vivian's doctor told her?
- What might Jesus say to Vivian?

Help us to remember, O God of Life, that acceptance of death is not the same as failure of faith. Remind us always of the life that is triumphant. Amen.

TONIGHT, I LEFT my son, Josh, at his college in Boston where he will begin his freshman year tomorrow. To say it was one of the hardest things I have ever done is an understatement. In fact, the thought I had—incredible as it may seem—is that it was easier to lose my breast than to let go of my son! Perhaps it is because my breast wasn't really an important part of my identity, whereas being a mother on an everyday basis is. Now it will be different—just as life without a left breast is different. Over time, it heals, the scar fades, and it simply becomes the way it is—a gentle reminder of something that once was whole and now is changed, never to be the same . . . the breast that covered and protected my heart.

- Have you ever had to let go of someone important as a part of life's transitions?
- How are you different as a result?
- What does our faith tell us about scars, healing, and wholeness?

Allow us the grace, our God, to say good-byes to the portions of life we cannot hold, and to open ourselves to greet that which is yet to come. Amen.

SOMETIMES, IT'S TRUE; there's just "no place like home"! After leaving Josh at college, I had arranged, with Richard's help, to catch a plane to the Twin Cities to be with my "other son." My only brother, Dan, is twelve years younger. Because of the age difference, he was almost like a "son" to me. I helped raise him, as my parents worked a lot. Instinctively, I knew I needed to be with him, and other family and old friends, in order to bridge the emotional gap of leaving Josh. How right this was! Being "home" was like balm for my soul—a true balm in Gilead, as the song says.

· Where do you go when you need to "go home"?
· Who are the family and friends you need to help you "bridge the gaps" in your life?
· Where is God in all of this?

Grant us, O God, a way to go to the home where we felt most safe and secure: to be in touch within our souls with those places and people and times that enrich and heal us. Whether it is within our power to be "there" in person, or if the blessing of imaginative prayer is what we must use, grant us the peace to make the journey. Amen.

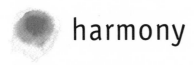

10

harmony

THIS SEEMS TO BE a period of starting new things for me. A time of rebirth. Thank God! When I moved here, I knew I wanted to start in Spiritual Direction (even though I wasn't entirely certain what it was). Over the years, I've had so very much psychotherapy and believed I needed to refocus my journey of self-discovery in a more spiritual direction. Thus, I was glad to find out that there was a retreat center near me that provided this. After my initial intake interview, however, I waited to be contacted for several months. Finally, I called to inquire if I had "failed the test" and to reiterate that I really wanted to pursue this avenue — and soon. Soon after this call, I began working weekly with a Spiritual Director. It took two tries to find the "right match." My Spiritual Director, Suzanne, is a warm, sensitive, and wise woman who really "hears" me. She is also a cancer survivor. I know intuitively that this is the right path for me — and that it needed to wait until now. God's perfect timing!

· Where do you see yourself spiritually at present?
· How do you deal with being "put off" or delayed when you're ready to begin something?
· Can you look at the role that "God's perfect timing" plays in your life? your illness?

Open to us new roads today, God. Give us new paths to walk on our journey to you, and fill us with the strength to take…just the next step. Amen.

ONE OF THE MORE enjoyable parts of our ministry to the community is on one evening a month when we meet with residents of a local nursing home. Richard does a mini-sermon, I sing a solo, and then we all sing old time hymns accompanied by Don, the Chaplain of Nursing Home Ministries and a marvelously gifted pianist. Some of the residents don't seem to be tracking at times but when the familiar gospel songs begin so does new life in them. The words flow from memory—often in childlike voices with tears or smiles of recognition. When Richard speaks, there are quite a few "Amens!" When Don rolls his arpeggios, there is joyful clapping. And when I sing, you can hear a pin drop. Whenever I sing, I try to prepare them with a few comments about why I chose a particular piece. Tonight I sang "On Eagle's Wings" by Michael Joncas, beginning by sharing my recent cancer recurrence with them. They were very attentive and quiet, then quickly followed with comments of caring and concern for us. I am incredulous, moved by their words and their presence. These are people that have been, in some cases, dismissed as "gone" or "useless" by others—but not at all! I am reminded how God sees none of us as beyond redemption—and how we are called to do the same for one another.

· Have you had experiences in nursing homes? How were they?
· What effect, if any, do the old gospel hymns have on you or others you've known? Do you have a favorite? (Pause a minute and sing it— gustily—aloud to yourself!)
· Imagine yourself being viewed as "old and useless" by others. What might this be like?

Let us not give up on ourselves, on each other, on those whom the world has pushed aside. Remind us of the preciousness and value of every moment of every life. Amen.

SOMETIMES I FORGET that I am not really an orphan in this world. I have been "adopted," once again, by another family— my husband Richard's family. It, like my own, is small and geo- graphically distant. He has one sister, Diana, a brother-in-law, Jerry, two nieces, Kelly and Kristin, and his mom, Wilma, all of whom live in the San Diego area. They have accepted me very much as one of them even though I am a second wife and not the mother of Richard's two children. When my mom died in February, Wilma said she'd like it if I called her "Mom" now— but only if I wanted to. Diana has taken to calling every Tuesday morning since we're both early risers. She always begins by say- ing, "This is your sister . . ." Jerry has sent me numerous articles on cancer and health. The nieces keep me plied with notes and e-mail to "Aunt Melody." It all helps more than they realize— just to be someone special in the lives of a group called "family." I often wonder how God keeps us all straight—such a large, di- verse family—and loves each of us through all the ups and downs of our lives. Amazing grace, is it not?

- What role have in-laws played in your life? In your illness? What pre- vents you from really becoming "family" to one another?
- Are there other groups in your life whom you call "family"? Who are these?
- Do you believe we're all equally children of God? Reflect on what it means to be a part of this Family . . .

Children of God . . . it has such a good sound. Grant us new opportunities to know our sisters and brothers, mothers and fathers, cousins and uncles and all. Put us in touch with your family again. Amen.

IF ANYONE EVER TOLD ME I'd be a stepmother someday, I'd have objected vehemently. "That is a role I'd never wish on my worst enemy," I'd have said, having counseled numerous stepfamilies in crisis. And yet, I fell in love with a man with two half-grown children, ages eight and twelve—and I one child, age five—and we soon wed. To varying degrees, all of our children have been opposed to our marriage—and each had his or her own ways of letting us know. But that was ten years ago and we have weathered the domestic storms—by the grace of God and some pretty skilled counselors. We've moved from survival mode to building a blended family identity (though, in truth, one never really "blends"). This time when I got sick, I had tearful loving calls from both stepkids—now grown and living back in California. Their support and caring was genuine and very touching to me. It all adds to my determination to stay alive for a good, long while. For one thing—and I don't want to rush them because neither of them is ready—I sure look forward to becoming a grandmother one day. And, believe me, there will be no "step" about it!

· What is your image of a stepmother? Do you have personal experience?

· Have you ever fallen in love with a person only to discover "it's a package deal"? How has this been for you?

· What do you think about words like "step" or "illegitimate"? How do they make you feel, thinking of them applied to yourself?

God of orphans and widows, of disgraced sisters and "illegitimate" sons, of refugees and remnants: blend us, we pray, into your family of faith and peace. Amen.

BEING HALF CHINESE, I have always been open to Eastern medicine. My father used to take me to Chinese herbalist shops—Asian pharmacies—when I was a kid. I remember them smelling odd but not unpleasant. This time when I have my recurrence, I have already been studying Tai-Chi off and on for a year. My doctor tells me I need to stop for now until the bones get stronger—so that is another loss. Wonderfully, one of my kindred spirits at church, Gini Bain, brings me literature on Chinese herbal medicines and introduces me to her practitioner. She does this with some trepidation—worried that I will find her "pushy" or him a "quack"—but I am delighted. After a consult and an exam, he places me on various combinations of herbs, which restore balance to my system. After a few visits, I decide to switch to Master Tom Tam, a Chinese healer, as I feel more true healing in his touch and presence. His office is in Boston, but we gladly make the trek because it fells right and good. My oncologist is supportive and interested. I feel blessed from both east and west!

- Do you have an experience of alternative or traditional folk medicine from your growing up? Is there a place for it in your current treatment?
- Have you ever been approached by someone like Gini? What was your reaction?
- Write down things you've thought of trying but haven't yet (for whatever reason).

Source of all truth and healing, we give you thanks for the blessings we share through and in spite of our differences. Amen.

THE MINISTERIAL ASSOCIATION IN OUR TOWN of Bloomfield had a daylong Good Friday service this year. Based on the Seven Last Words of Christ, it featured seven different preachers with special music from each of their churches. When it was our turn, my husband spoke—well, as always. After this, I sang a duet with a new friend, Renata DiPietro. The song was "Pie Jesu" from *Requiem* by Andrew Lloyd Weber, a beautiful, haunting piece. I sang the boy soprano part and Renata, a gifted professional, the operatic soprano. People were enthralled by the music and the blend of our two voices; it was truly a holy moment. What struck me was the fact that such beautiful music came from two women both struggling with serious health issues: Renata is a diabetic who is legally blind, I a three-time cancer survivor.

· What style of preaching moves you most? Can you recall a particular preacher, sermon, or service that reached you?
· Is there a piece of sacred music that gives you a sense of the "holy"? Any idea why?
· Make time to listen to that piece this week and reflect here …

Let your Perfect Love flow through all of us, imperfect vessels that we are. Let the content of your grace be the focus of our faith. Amen.

FROM AGE FIVE, I took piano lessons until I was about twelve. My teacher, Miss Sunday, a very serious and somewhat scary spinster lady, thought I had "promise." That was all my mother, a lover of music, needed to hear. I, however much talent I had, possessed little discipline and practiced as little as possible, thus making little progress. Yet, as an adult, I find myself drawn back to the piano, especially now that I can no longer sing. At a recent party, friends were jamming and I was moved to the keyboard by a wise three-year-old boy who wanted me to play the keys next to him. How could he have intuited that it was exactly what I needed to do?

· What role have music lessons played in your life?
· If you could express yourself musically, what form would it take?
· Do you believe God can call to us through a three-year-old?

From the fingers of babes hast thou brought forth perfect praise. Is even imperfect praise acceptable to you, God? Amen.

TODAY WAS GREAT FUN! Brother Dan, two young women from his church, Crystal and Heather, and I went to the Minnesota State Fair. Now, I can say without bias that this is the best state fair in the country. Our parents used to have Chinese food concessions there at which I worked every summer, so I know it very well. Fortunately, it has not changed a lot since then. (Some things ought to stay the same, in my opinion!) We had much enjoyment just walking around, checking out the people and the exhibits, sampling lots of unhealthy but tasty foods, spending money on the games (at which my brother won five stuffed animals!), and taking some midway rides. What a treat for all the senses, especially the memory!

· Do you have a tradition, like the State Fair, that you still enjoy?
· What is your favorite part of this experience?
· Can you recall the last time you participated in something like this, just acting like a kid out for a good time?

God of apple pies and big stuffed teddies, of ferris wheels and blue-ribbon calves: remind us, or recall us, to the simple celebrations of simple life. Bless us with naivete, if only for this day. Amen.

ONE OF MY MAIN PURPOSES in going home was to get to see my aunties, my mom's three sisters, of whom I have written elsewhere. They were so close to my mom—an inseparable foursome—and such a regular part of our growing up. The cousins, of whom there are a dozen, were like a large, extended family, spending most holidays and many summers at our lake cabin. So I was thrilled that I was able to see all three aunties, the two remaining uncles, and four of my cousins as well as one of their kids. It felt like a real reunion! We prayed, ate, laughed, reminisced, and even cried a little. It was so precious to have one uncle say, "You're just as obstreperous as ever, Melody!" and the other one remark, "You don't change a bit—you look like a girl!" The aunties all spoke lovingly to us, one saying to me, "I loved you the minute I saw you and it's never changed, honey . . ." The cousins all exchanged e-mail addresses and hugs in saying our good-byes.

· What role does extended family play in your life?
· How have they related to your illness?
· Do you experience the love of God in your family gatherings? If not, what can you do to bring this about?

God of all our families, of brothers and sisters and aunties all: celebrate with us those joys of reunion and remembrance, that we might know how precious we (still) are. Amen.

I HAVE SOME long-term relationships that aren't easy to define in traditional terms. One of these is with Sheila, who lived with our family for several years. Her mom and mine were best friends—like sisters—and her dad and mine "shirttail relations," so we joke that we are sisters, cousins, and friends—and let other people try to figure it out! As we've grown older, we've gotten closer as a result of sharing so many life experiences in common. Like me, Sheila had her only child in her thirties, two months before me, married a man with half-grown kids, and gave up a lucrative career to follow her heart. This trip, we shared the recent experience of leaving our kids at college. We also shared about getting older and how that feels to each of us. However, the thing that gave us the most energy and joy was the possibility of Sheila, an accomplished graphic designer, doing the cover and layout for this book. She pored over my meditations and I over her portfolio until we discovered common ground on which to build. The result is the lovely watercolor that graces the cover of this book.

- Is there a "Sheila" in your life, someone who defies categorization but is undeniably significant in your life?
- Think of someone whose life experiences more or less mirror your own and write that person a letter.
- Do you think God is a part of the coming together in the creative process?

"Who are my mother, and sisters, and brothers? Those who do God's will." We who are related to you through one another, and through one another to you, pray that your creative will be done. Amen.

A FAMILIAR REFRAIN from a song we used to sing in Brownies goes, "Make new friends, but keep the old; One is silver and the other gold." The older I get, the more I realize the profound truth in this simple song. Not that new friends are any less precious, but old friends are much like gold in that the friendship has been refined over the years. Today I got to spend six blessed hours with Sandy and Linda, friends since kindergarten. They always make time for me when I come to town—no questions asked—and I always leave feeling connected and "filled up" by them. Because we have known one another so long, we need no preambles or excuses. We simply get into being with one another. It is easy and comfortable. The time passes gently and quickly. They are true gifts from God!

- How do you feel about the lyrics from this song?
- Do you have friends like Sandy and Linda who "knew you when" and love you now?
- Can you sense God's presence in your friendships?

For the gifts of childhood that grow older along with us, we are grateful, loving God. Enable us to renew and nurture and treasure those who are still children with us. Amen.

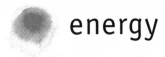

energy

IT IS MY HUSBAND Richard's day off (if, in fact, that can ever truly be said of pastors!), so we decide to take a road trip. We take along our dog Sam—a true "angel" in canine form according to all who meet him. He loves to travel—no matter where or when—and always has a sense of excitement and adventure about any journey. He's even happy to go on errands and stay in the car in the parking lot; after all, one never knows what could happen. At the bank drive-up window, he even gets a dog biscuit! Today, I really need to borrow from his enthusiasm because mine is waning, as is my energy after my first week of radiation. Richard is also upbeat—"One down, two to go!"—and he loves driving as much as Sam does riding. However, even their "joie de vivre" is not enough to keep me awake and I soon drift off to sleep. Upon awakening, I am upset with myself for missing the scenery, but my husband is happy I rested and my dog is glad just to have me back. Amazingly, I realize they both love me just the way I am—and only want me to feel better. God's love in human (and canine) form!

· Is there someone around you who is willing and able to "lend" you some energy or enthusiasm when yours flags (as it will)?

- How can you be more attuned to your need for "down time" and learn to honor it?
- Are there "creatures" in your life who comfort and care for you? Write a letter of thanks to them here and then find some way to let them know how grateful you are for their presence …

Let us be loved by you today, O God: in whatever disguise you appear. Amen.

WHAT A GLORIOUS DAY this was! Truly "a feast for all the senses"! During the morning worship service, several of us choir members presented a cantata. It was kind of risky because it was contemporary rock music accompanied by keyboard, guitar, and drums —in the sanctuary, no less. There were times we even danced and clapped! Thank God, the congregation joined us in the joy of it all. (Who says New England Congregationalists have to be uptight?) After that, we went to brunch to celebrate our debut together. Soon we were back at church getting ready to serve fifty parishioners at our first annual Pastor's Pentecost "Tongues of Fire" Pasta Party. Lots of good, spicy food and fellowship. At one point, while I was scurrying from kitchen to dining room, one of the ladies touched me gently on the arm and asked, "Now—are you doing too much to tire yourself, Melody?" I was touched by her compassion and surprised that I had not even thought about my cancer all day. How good it was to be cared for enough so that I could care for others! The circle of compassion—all of us held together by God's loving arms, encircling us, feeding and renewing body, mind, and spirit. Setting us on fire!

- Have you ever been to a feast? Describe what this was like with every sense you can …
- What is the mood in your church, synagogue, temple, or faith community when you gather for worship and fellowship?
- How do you feel when people reach out to you in compassion and concern?

Thank you, God, for the circles of love, tongues of fire, and breaths of the Spirit that bind us to one another and give power to our compassion and love. Amen.

THIS MORNING, a good friend from Iowa called: Renee, a creative, quirky, and engaging artist. Renee helped me tremendously at a time when I felt abused and rejected. Her quick wit and wisdom could see the humor and meaning even in dark times. One of her gifts to me was a little book entitled *Don't Sweat the Small Stuff . . . and it's all Small Stuff!* Our life in Iowa, particularly our church experience, was anything but positive. Yet, nothing is without some redeeming aspects and this friendship was surely redemptive. She has encouraged me to let go of the hurtful past and to move beyond it to a more hopeful future. I know she's right—but I still find myself caught at times between the two, in a present that, at best, can be called "bittersweet." Why is this? I believe it has to do with long being stuck between self-righteous anger and life-giving forgiveness (so I'm human!). I know that in order to get well and stay well, I need to "let go and let God," the Alcoholics Anonymous (AA) credo. Yet, in my humanness, I hang on despite my desire to let go. I am comforted by remembering

Jesus' struggle with the mean, deceitful people in his life, how he had to pray, asking God to forgive—perhaps because, in his humanity, he could not.

· How has humor or "quirkiness" helped you cope with your illness? If it hasn't, why not?
· What is some of the "small stuff" you might be "sweating"? Make a list here …
· Take your list and, each day, for as many days as it takes, pray for forgiveness—letting go—of that item …

Grant us, O God, the forgiveness of others. Amen.

SINCE WE'VE MOVED, I've rediscovered the—for me—lost art of letter writing. This has been fostered, in part, by my love of receiving mail! Ever since I can remember, I have waited excitedly for the mail to arrive. Maybe, just maybe, there'll be something in it today for me . . . I mean, besides bills and ads! My precious friend Kathi has been the most faithful in keeping a correspondence going with me. When I receive a letter from her, I know it will be full of both news and good wishes to keep me updated and filled up. Kathi is a healer—a social worker by trade—and she is without a doubt the most affirming and accepting person I have ever known. And she is my friend—a fact that makes me feel incredibly blessed. I look forward to the giving and receiving that has become a tangible sign of our deep, abiding connection. Keep those cards and letters coming . . . with an occasional phone call just so I can laugh with you over nothing in particular, dearest friend, except the joy of our friendship.

· Do you like getting personal letters? What about writing them? What is the best letter you ever received?

· Write a letter to someone you've been meaning to, someone who's been on your mind and in your heart (whether or not you "owe" them a letter!).

· Yes—write a letter to God! It might help to think of it as a "prayer on paper."

Give us the time today, God, to read some of your Word, and to write a letter back to you. Let this be a renewal of our regular communication with you. Amen.

ONE OF THE GREATEST things about moving is the chance to get to make new friends. A couple moves ago, I had decided not to get close to anyone because I knew we'd only be there a short time . . . what a mistake that was! This time, the person I met first—a neighbor and a church member—is proving to be my newest "best friend." Carol is a soul sister in so many ways; we are both small of stature but big on energy and enthusiasm. Anything goes: we take walks and talk, go on road trips, pick berries and make jam, plan and plant gardens, practice our Tai Chi moves and laugh at one another! She is my "whatever" friend—a friend in whatever circumstance, large or small. She has helped me in more ways than she could ever know, and we're only just beginning. I am reminded again of a song from Girl Scout days that reminds me of us: "Make new friends, but keep the old; one is silver and the other gold!" I think Carol and I will move over the years from silver to gold.

- Recall a time when you moved that was especially difficult for you. What made it so hard?
- How do you go about making friends? What do you look for and value in a friendship? Write a want ad for a friend: i.e., "Wanted: Friend …"
- Describe yourself as a friend. Make a "personal" ad asking people to consider being your friend.

Today, O God, let me be open to finding—and becoming—a new friend. Let me gain the strength that comes from such growth. Amen.

12

unity

SOMETHING HAPPENED yesterday after God finally got through to me—because I'm actually finding myself looking forward to my treatments. Not that I enjoy the process of being "zapped" as I call it, but I enjoy my developing connections with other patients in the waiting room. There are several of us who keep showing up, morning after morning, at about the same time. So, we are starting to get to know one another beyond just the superficial conversational gambits. There's something about sitting in a waiting room in a hospital gown and stocking feet that takes away all the artificial barriers and distinctions. We are all just people— wounded, vulnerable, frightened, but, above all, hopeful—and it is a bond that goes deep to where God dwells in each of us.

· Have you been able to connect with others going through the same experience? How has this been for you? Would you like more of this? What could help it to happen?
· What kinds of masks or disguises might you be wearing to "get by"?
· Try to imagine what it would be like to remove these and just be yourself ...

Enable us today to see past the masks and disguises to the real people in our lives. Empower us to take away the masks and disguises that are our own. Amen.

ONE OF THE HOSPICE NURSES, Carline, and I attend a seventy-ninth birthday party for E. She has breast cancer that has spread to the brain—not a good prognosis. In fact, no one thought she'd be alive this long (except E. herself—she just knew it!). The party is held at her favorite local restaurant. There are so many guests that we take up a large back room by ourselves. E. is sitting in the place of honor, surrounded by friends and gifts, looking pretty and happy. She greets each of us in turn with smiles and hugs and introduces us all around. I am honored when she pats the seat next to her for me to take. After all, I am not "family" and have probably known her the shortest amount of time. In a flash, I realize she's most likely doing this to make me feel comfortable. She's taking care of me! I feel humbled by this knowledge and grateful for her compassion. We are, after all, travelers on the same road, she and I. One of us may simply get there before the other one. There is no real difference between us—certainly not to God, anyway.

- When is the last time you felt "special" in a crowd? What was this like for you?
- Do you have a relationship with anyone right now of "mutual care"?
- Plan a "party" for yourself. Describe it here . . .

Hold us all in your cupped hands of care, O God. Let us lose track of who is the caregiver, who the cared for. Let us all simply and clearly know that our caring is in truth a part of yours. Amen.

I MUST BE one of the only persons I know who gains weight when I have cancer—every time! I've always had a cast-iron stomach and nothing affects my appetite (not even chemotherapy). Oh well! However, one of the side effects of not having much energy is that I didn't do my normal walking and wasn't allowed to play tennis. As a result, I got kind of flabby, to put it bluntly but truthfully. (They say honesty is the first step in AA . . .) So I joined the local Jewish Community Center, and today I started back to aqua-aerobics. And what a pleasure it was! There is something so elemental about being in the water. I feel more in touch with my "child" self and lighter because of the buoyancy factor. I can do things I wouldn't be able to ever do on land. Plus it is so much fun to bounce around in the water, laughing and talking with a pool full of other people of all types, ages, and sizes. We are kids, in a big bathtub, being cleansed and rejuvenated, and all of us are children of God! I was rather tired afterward but it was a good tired. I know it will get easier the more I stay with it. For now, I'm just thankful for new beginnings. Not surprisingly, I met another woman, Ann, also a social worker, who is undergoing radiation treatments. What else? I feel we will become friends. What a bonus!

· How has your body changed in the process of living with cancer? How do you feel about it?
· Reflect on the importance of water to a child (bathing, swimming, etc.). See if you can recall incidents from your childhood and how this differs from adulthood.
· What might you like to do to get yourself "in shape" again? What keeps you from doing this?

We move through the Spirit of God like fish in the ocean, or birds in the air. Remind us again of this, O God. Amen.

People often remind me of animals—mostly dogs, as they are my favorite four-legged creatures. Sometimes, while walking my dog, I amuse myself by noticing how much owners and their dogs come to resemble one another. Then I remind myself that my dog is brown, overweight, and overly friendly! My radiologist, whom I will call Dr. Jeff Steinberg, brings to mind a cuddly, aging mutt. He is short, balding (probably from all the pats on the head he's received!) and very sweet-natured. It is obvious that he's been well-loved and cared for by the way he returns this to his patients. He listens intently with his big, brown, puppy-dog eyes full of gentleness and compassion. They say that eyes are the window to one's soul—and the soul is definitely at home in this kindly Jewish doctor.

· What do you think of my notion that dogs and their owners resemble one another?
· Do you have a dog (or cat—or whatever) and how has this creature helped you during your illness?
· Does your dog resemble you? (Be honest—and smile at the realization, if you're able!)

We praise you, O God, for the diversity of creation, for the divine in the human, for the "human" in the "canine," for life in all its wonder. Amen.

MY FRIENDS TEASE ME about being a "church lady"—and I guess I am. Since coming to Bloomfield, I've become involved with Church Women United, an ecumenical international organization of dedicated "church ladies." A lot of the women in our unit are older, many of them African American, all of them warm and welcoming to me, calling me "young lady"! When they talk about their faith, it feels deep and real—tangible in their faces and voices. One of our projects this summer was to make quilts to send to African women and children. It was in the making of these quilts—ironing, designing, cutting, and stitching—that we showed ourselves to one another. Their love and concern for me was both fussy and comforting, much like that of my mom and aunties when I was growing up in Minnesota. They inquired each time we met, with genuine interest, ". . . and how are you doing, dear?" The quilts became, for me, a symbol of our mingled creativity—all colors and patterns coming together to make something warm and nurturing from one woman to all women . . .

· Do you see yourself as a "church lady" (or man)? What does this term convey to you?
· Are there opportunities in your life to be with people of different ages, faiths, and races? If not, would you like there to be?
· If your life were a quilt, what would it look like (in words or images)?

Bind us to one another, God, and make of our togetherness more beauty than we can imagine. Show us that unity and diversity can truly be wonderful. Amen.

ONE OF THE WOMEN I have met from Church Women United, Debbie, has become a role model for me of the kind of mature Christian woman I would like to become. In my mind, I have fantasized asking her to be my mentor in the faith—but I haven't yet found the courage to actually do so. It isn't so much that she's a leader; rather, it's how she leads: in gentleness and firmness of conviction. Her life is one of faith-in-action in a true UCC fashion. One of the ways in which she has touched me during my illness is to take an active part in helping to sell Angels of Hope pins. These are made by the Guatemalan Women's Co-op to support themselves and their children in this war-ravaged country. Debbie has taken the pins with her to many meetings all over the country. Today, she left me an envelope with a check and a note saying "praying for you . . ." Through her efforts, I feel I am helping even when I myself am not the one doing the work . . . the sisterhood of Christ!

· Do you have a role model for the person you'd like to become?
· In what ways do you "put your faith in action"?
· How do you feel when someone says "I'm praying for you …"?

For strengthening our faith by adding it to the faithfulness of others, we give you thanks, O God. Help us together to do your will. Amen.

LORALEE IS ONE of the first friends I made at the church after we moved here. This was initially due to her continually reaching out to me via cards, calls, and invitations to become involved. Her care was sincere and heartfelt and it sparked a chord in me. She is also one of the most eclectic persons I know—always learning and studying something new and challenging (Old Testament Greek was her latest venture!). This weekend brought a new challenge to our friendship. We attended a UCC Women's Celebration in Portland, Maine, and roomed together. In my experience, this is one of the quickest—and scariest—ways to test a friendship. We found that we are very different from one another in our little daily habits: Loralee's very slow, methodical, and neat in her ways while I'm "quick and dirty" in mine. She's usually late and I'm always running to be just on time. Yet we managed to laugh about these differences and began to call one another "big and little sister."

· Who has reached out to you in a time of transition? During this time of illness?
· Have you had the experience of rooming with someone quite different from yourself?
· Do you have big or little "sisters"? (family or friends) Have you let them know their importance in your life? If not, do so here …

We celebrate, O God, the diversity that brings you such joy in creation; we rejoice in our delightful differences. Amen.

THE NEW ENGLAND UCC Women's Conference in Portland, Maine, was entitled "Celebration," and indeed it was! The worship and workshops were inspirational and informative. The camaraderie and communication were fun and meaningful. But, for me, the best part is almost always the music, and this was no exception. Singing sacred music in a group of two thousand women moves me beyond words. It is as if I am transported to the heart of God. This morning, when we were singing in worship, a woman seated next to me turned and said, "You sing like an angel—and you look like one, too. Your name suits you perfectly." I was astounded—touched and humbled. How could it be, I wondered, that she could see this in one who is fighting for her life right now?

· Have you ever attended an event like "Celebration"? Write some adjectives here describing it.
· Do you like to sing? What is it like for you? Have you ever sung in such a large gathering?
· What about this image of "being transported to the heart of God"? Can you relate to it?
· Do you ever feel surprised when people see the health and wholeness in you at this time?

Help us, dear Lord, to allow the light of your love to shine not just in our darkened moments, but through them, as well. Amen.

AFTER CHURCH ON SUNDAY, I spot a very striking gray-haired black man standing by himself at coffee hour. When I introduce myself, I am pleased to discover John Akeife, a preacher from Ghana, who has come to visit his son who lives nearby. He has been attending various churches in the area, seeking to build alliances between his country and ours, so I introduce him to Richard. For the next several weeks that he is here, he attends regularly and they speak often. One of their joint projects is to secure Bibles for him to bring back with him when he returns to his country. Before he leaves, he gives Richard a tie and me a stole, both with symbols of Ghana. He tells me that all minister's wives are called "mama" in his country. I like this! Richard gives John a communion chalice from his set to take back with him, and John cries. We have all been profoundly touched by our brief contact with one another.

· Have you had any contact with folks from other cultures? How has this been for you? And how do you think it was for them?
· Think about how simple requests—like Bibles—can mean so much. Are there any small ways in your life you could be an "ambassador" to someone from another country?
· What mementos do you cherish from other places? Why?

Remind us, God of all Creation, of our oneness with one another around your world. Help us be open to new opportunities to be brother or sister to a "stranger." Amen.

ONE OF THE GAMES I have wanted to learn since childhood is mah-jongg. I used to love to watch the Chinese ladies playing, clicking tiles and chattering away in Cantonese. I inherited a handcarved ivory set that my father brought from China as a boy. This spring, I had the chance to take a class at our local Senior Center. Actually, I talked my way in, as I am "only fifty-three" but am a member of the Commission on Aging for our town. Hannah, our teacher, tickled me when she said I was a "fast learner." I responded, "I ought to be; I'm at least twenty years younger than the rest of you." Hannah and most of the players are in their seventies and eighties, many of them Jewish, with a couple of Catholics, and me, the lone Protestant. Truly an ecumenical gathering of women! I have made connections over the clicking tiles with Tina, Helen, and Hyla. We meet in one another's homes to play weekly as well. I so look forward to my mah-jongg days that I schedule my doctor appointments around them!

· Do you have an ethnic game or activity you play or would like to?
· Are there places in your life for intergenerational gatherings?
· Is there ecumenism?

God beyond the limits of our beliefs, be present to us in the diversity of others, and in the diversion of play. Amen.

AS LIFE WOULD HAVE IT, I have had two "cancer partners" with which to share this experience intimately. Both of them are close friends, one from Iowa and one from Connecticut. Gloria has a particularly aggressive form of breast cancer and has been in almost constant treatment since it was diagnosed recently. Vivian has lived with cancer for twenty-five years. It is now in her liver, for which she is now receiving palliative treatments. Glo and I have an e-mail correspondance; Viv and I speak on the phone regularly. Much of our conversations revolve around each of our struggles with this dreadful disease and how it is affecting us and those we love. It is a relief to be able to have contact with someone to whom one need not explain or be protective but rather simply let it all hang out—for good or ill. We often end up crying or laughing together, sometimes at the same moment. The words and feelings expressed by one of us could well be said by the other. I always end a communication with either of them emptied and filled up at the same time. That is why I was so surprised when each of them, independent of the other (because they have not met, although they would become fast friends, of that I am sure), said basically the same thing to me. Glo wrote how "upbeat and hopeful" I always am and Viv remarked how I always "lift her spirits." This was quite a shock to me, as I have felt I was often a downer with both of them!

· Have you been surprised to hear how others see you during this illness?
· Do you have folks like Glo and Viv with whom you can really be yourself?
· What part do you think God plays in these relationships?

God, be our partner . . . in the pain . . . in the possibility . . . in the promise. Amen.

OTHER BOOKS FROM THE PILGRIM PRESS

THE BOOK OF DAILY PRAYER, MORNING AND EVENING 2002
KIM MARTIN SADLER, EDITOR

A book of morning and evening devotionals for those who long for the nurture of a daily prayer life. Each prayer is written in the style of "praying the scripture." These prayers have ministered to all who read them.

0-8298-1413-2/376 pages/paper/$13.00

LIKE A SECOND LAYER OF SKIN
100 Affirmations for Faithful Living
DOROTHY WINBUSH RILEY

Like a Second Layer of Skin acknowledges the power within each of us to speak our lives into existence. By listening to ourselves speak positively and affirmatively, we have the opportunity to create the kind of spiritual environment in which we would want to live.

0-8298-1411-6/112 pages/paper/$10.00

DEEP IN THE FAMILIAR
Four Life Rhythms
JOAN CANNON BORTON

Using the four traditional Hindu life phrases—"Student," "Householder," "Time in the Forest," and "Return to the Village"—Borton has written a book that enables women to explore their life's path with an awareness of these life phrases or "rhythms." Through this process, women can become more fully awake to the sacred nature of their daily lives.

0-8298-1408-6/208 pages/paper/$16.00

To order call THE PILGRIM PRESS
1-800-537-3394